What Women Want To Know About BREAST IMPLANTS

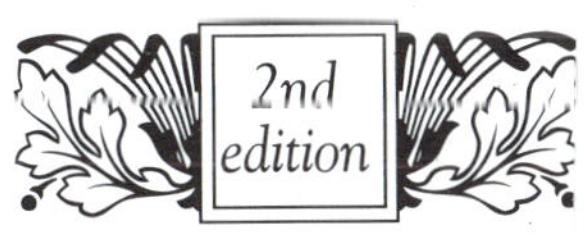

2nd edition

AF334499

Karen Berger and John Bostwick III, M.D.

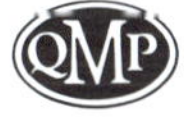

Quality Medical Publishing, Inc.

ST. LOUIS, MISSOURI
1998

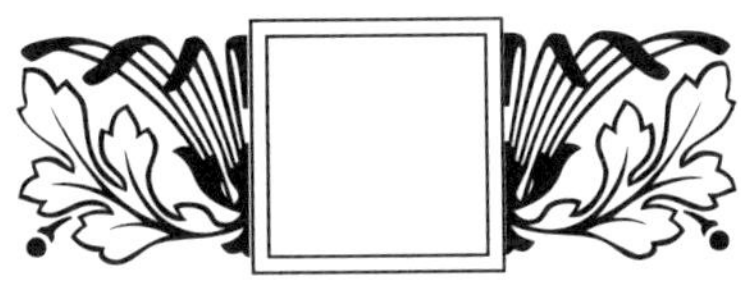

WHAT WOMEN WANT TO KNOW ABOUT BREAST IMPLANTS

Breast implants have been an integral part of breast surgery for almost 35 years. They have been successfully used to restore breast shape and contour after mastectomy, correct breast and chest wall deformities and asymmetries, augment small breasts, and lift sagging ones. Although the efficacy of these devices is widely recognized and acknowledged, in recent years major concerns have arisen about their safety. The intense media coverage of the so-called implant controversy and the Food and Drug Administration (FDA) restrictions on implant availability pending further research heightened public concern. Emotions often triumphed over logic. Today, however, with the passage of time and after numerous scientific studies, this topic can be approached with a fresh perspective. Questions about safety are being fully addressed, the hysteria has largely dissipated, and the breast implant story is no longer front-page news. The scientific facts can stand on their own merit. Recent clinical studies have assuaged earlier fears, allowing these devices to be judged impartially based on the scientific data accumulated.

The following discussion attempts to address women's questions and concerns, to present the facts, to review the latest scientific studies, and to put this topic into perspective so that women can judge for themselves. The majority of this discussion is devoted to questions that women want answered. These queries are those posed by women in personal interviews and surveys. The answers are based on published medical studies and reports, data supplied by experts, and current documented scientific evidence. Unlike the anecdotal reports of individual patients often featured in the media, these scientifically controlled studies compare women with and without implants. The latter group of women, called a *control group,* serves to determine whether health problems in those with implants are occurring more frequently than might be expected in the general population.

We begin by discussing the benefits and risks of these devices.

What is the value of breast implants?

Breast implants were originally developed in the early 1960s for women who desired breast enhancement. Some of these women's breasts became smaller after pregnancy, and they wanted their breasts to be fuller once again; others thought their breasts were too small, poorly formed, or out of proportion to their total body shape. Implants offered a viable and effective solution to their problems. Building on patient satisfaction with implant surgery for breast enlargement, surgeons soon recognized that these devices were also well suited for restoring breast shape and contour after mastectomy for breast cancer and for correcting breast and chest wall asymmetries and congenital chest wall deformities.

Since the introduction of implants almost 35 years ago, approximately 1 million women in the United States have had breast implant surgery. Implants have made a difference to these women. They have offered a return to normalcy for women with breast cancer and an opportunity to put the cancer experience behind them and get on with their lives. Breast reconstruction has helped these women to feel whole again; they have reported feeling good about themselves once again, with renewed self-confidence and a new zest for life. Still others say that implants have provided them with a more normal body image, a more flattering breast form, or an improved self-image. The benefits of breast implants have been both physical and psychological, and their value for women's health has become more obvious with time. Many cancer specialists believe and our experience would suggest that knowing that breast reconstruction is an option will save many women's lives because they will not procrastinate in seeking care for breast problems for fear of breast loss.

What are the psychological benefits of breast implants?

Since breast implants are used to enhance small breasts and reconstruct breasts after mastectomy, the benefit is primarily psychological. Women who have had breast implants report that their self-esteem is enhanced—that they feel more attractive, less self-conscious, more feminine, and more self-confident. Women who have had implants for breast reconstruction report that they no longer feel deformed as they did following mastectomy; they feel more normal and less depressed over their appearance. Most describe a restored sense of well-being and relief at not having a "constant reminder of their cancer and mortality."

What are the physical benefits of implants?

Implants can be used to correct breast or chest wall asymmetries associated with developmental conditions or trauma. They are also used for breast reconstruction after mastectomy. Many women who have had mastectomies report that the implant helps restore a feeling of balance. For women with a large opposite breast, it may also alleviate back and shoulder pain and postural problems caused by attempts to disguise the uneven chest with a heavy external prosthesis. The implant can provide cover for the exposed chest wall, which may be sensitive after breast removal. It can also be used to replace an external prosthesis, thereby affording a woman greater freedom in selecting clothing styles and avoiding the discomfort and skin irritation that sometime accompany use of an external breast prosthesis.

What is the reported satisfaction rate of women who have had implant surgery?

A number of studies have been done to assess the satisfaction rate after breast implant operations. These studies have shown that over 60% and sometimes as many as 80% to 90% of the women who have had implant surgery for augmentation are pleased with the results of the procedure. Approximately 94% of these women reported that the results of augmentation met their expectations. A 1997 study involving 504 patients at 11 different centers adds further credence to these statistics, reporting overall patient satisfaction at 94.2% after surgery with saline-filled implants (usually for breast augmentation). Similar satisfaction rates have been reported with implant surgery for breast reconstruction; however, because skin may be thinner at the mastectomy site, the possibility of complications is higher for reconstructive procedures than for breast augmentation. Despite problems, most women say, and our surveys confirm, that they would choose to have implant surgery again.

What kind of breast implants are currently available? What type of fillings are used in them?

Basically there are two broad categories of implants: fixed-volume breast implants and implants in which the volume can be changed after they are implanted (tissue expanders). All of the currently available implants have an outer layer or envelope of silicone that is in contact with the body tissues. These implants are usually filled with saline (saltwater) solution. Silicone gel–filled implants are also available but only on a relatively limited basis in the United States.

Alternate filling materials for the implant envelopes are under investigation to determine if these materials are radiolucent, as opposed to opaque, and easily eliminated or removed by the body if they leak. These fillings will provide possible alternatives to those currently in use. Some of the fillings being investigated include water-based gels; gel-like solutions consisting of water, salts, and organic polymers; and purified soybean oil. Currently no breast implants with alternative fillings are commercially available in the United States. An implant that has a silicone shell filled with a purified soybean oil is presently being studied to determine whether mammograms can more effectively detect breast masses with this type of implant than with a silicone gel–filled or a saline-filled implant.

Implants are also available with smooth and with textured silicone surfaces. Many surgeons believe that these textured surfaces have helped to reduce the incidence of breast hardness (capsular contracture) after implant surgery. However, in some patients these textured-surface implants are more visible and may exhibit a rippled appearance through the skin.

How do the aesthetic results of operations with saline-filled implants compare to those achieved with silicone gel–filled implants?

Certain characteristics of silicone gel–filled breast implants make them preferable to saline-filled implants. The gel has a more natural consistency than saltwater and feels and flows more like a natural breast. These implants also offer flexibility in designing different breast shapes—some wider, some with additional projection to allow for individualization. Saline-filled implants are more limited in their shape; they are also slightly heavier than silicone gel–filled implants and when overfilled are firm, almost spherical, and therefore feel and look unnatural. When underfilled they can be soft, and their envelopes, which are generally thicker than those containing silicone gel, can develop noticeable and palpable folds and ripples, particularly through thin skin at the mastectomy site. Some of the newer models of saline implants have "shaped" contours that seem to help mini-

mize wrinkling problems and improve the contour of the reconstructed breast.

Is one brand or type of breast implant better or safer than another?

Although some surgeons have expressed "a higher level of comfort"
with the safety of saline-filled implants and others prefer a particular
type of implant because they have experienced more success with it,
for example, in avoiding certain adverse effects such as capsular contracture, it will not be known for certain whether one brand or model
is more effective than another until the FDA evaluates the safety and
effectiveness of all breast implants. Ongoing clinical trials are under-
way to evaluate silicone gel–filled implants. The formal review of the
safety and effectiveness of saline-filled implants began in 1993. The
information gathered by two U.S. manufacturers has already been
submitted to the FDA for evaluation. All preclinical data as well as
the deflation and complication rates will be submitted toward the end
of 1998.

Is silicone safe to use in humans?

Silicone, a commonly used substance for various implantable devices,
is considered by many to be one of the least reactive biomaterials. Initially introduced for evaluation in medical applications in the 1940s,
silicone is used for artificial joints, implantable pumps, shunts, drains,
ocular implants, and other devices that require a material that is relatively nonreactive, nonallergenic, and easily tolerated by the body.
Implantable silicone devices include pacemakers, hydrocephalus
shunts, breast implants, penile implants, and testicular implants. Anyone who has ever taken a capsule has probably ingested silicone, for it
is used to coat many capsules to make them more easily swallowed.
Silicone is also present in processed foods, in cosmetics, and in many
drugs (especially antacids). Silicone is used to lubricate syringes, in in-
travenous tubing, and in shunts used for chemotherapy. Anyone who
has had blood drawn or been given an injection has had some silicone
introduced into his or her body. Many infant pacifiers are made of silicone. As Dr. James Potchen, a radiologist at the University of Michigan explains, "Some systemic levels of silicone will be found in every
patient with an implant. The fact is that a very low level of silicone is
present in everyone. The relationship between use of insulin syringes

by diabetics and systemic levels of silicone is just as impressive as that in patients with implants that bleed." If silicone represents a serious chemical hazard to the human body, this should already be apparent because of this chemical's widespread use. The fact is it doesn't. Nevertheless, studies continue to rule out the possibility of currently unrecognized and rare problems. New silicone devices are routinely receiving FDA approval. For example, silicone oil, a new product for reattaching the retina in complicated cases of retinal detachment, has received FDA authorization to be marketed.

What problems are associated with implants and how often do they occur?

As with all devices, implants are not without problems. They are subject to local complications such as rupture, possible leakage, deflation, displacement, deformation, and capsular contracture, the latter being the most common problem. They also may interfere with mammograms and cause calcium deposits to accumulate in the capsule tissue that forms around implants. Breast implant surgery may cause changes in breast and nipple sensation. These problems are not life threatening, however, and are usually correctable.

One of our most accurate sources on the frequency of local complications is the unaudited 4-year results of the Mentor Adjunct Study (a cooperative effort between Mentor Corporation and the FDA). This study reports the incidence of capsular contracture and the occurrence of complications in 15,544 patients receiving silicone gel–filled breast implants. In this 5-year study the researchers reported capsular contracture rates as follows: 8.8% of patients experienced minimal contracture, 3.7% moderate, and 1.1% severe. The three most frequently cited complications were breast pain, implant wrinkling, and breast asymmetry. Interestingly, only a small percentage of patients (less than 1%) chose to have secondary surgery to have these problems corrected.

How do the risks associated with saline-filled implants compare to those associated with silicone gel–filled implants?

Shrinkage of the scar tissue (capsular contracture) and calcium deposit formation occur with both saline-filled and silicone gel–filled implants. Deflation of the implant may be more likely with the saline-filled type. When a saline-filled implant develops a leak, it is likely to deflate over a period of hours to days or even weeks, requiring surgical replacement within a month or two or when the implant has lost most of its volume and become flat. Some saline-filled implants will deflate spontaneously, losing all the saline solution at once and requiring re-operation for implant replacement.

Is there a special risk for women with polyurethane-coated implants?

In about 11% of women who had silicone gel–filled breast implants a type of implant coated with polyurethane foam was used. The coating was designed to reduce the incidence of capsular contracture. These implants are no longer available in the United States because the company manufacturing them has discontinued production.

The polyurethane coating can be chemically broken down under specific laboratory conditions to release tiny amounts of a substance called toluene diamine (TDA), which has been found to cause cancer in laboratory mice. It is not known whether the foam breaks down to TDA in the body; however, the FDA has determined that "it is unlikely that even one of the estimated 110,000 women who got polyurethane foam–covered implants will get cancer as a result of exposure to TDA." Studies using the latest tests to detect minute levels of TDA were conducted under FDA guidance and showed a slight increase in levels of TDA but no indication of an increased risk. According to the FDA, a woman's lifetime cancer risk, if any, is likely to be miniscule, about one in a million over a lifetime.

What is capsular contracture? Does this pose a serious risk for women who have implant surgery?

A capsule is firm, fibrous scar tissue that forms around a breast implant. This is a characteristic response of the body to isolate any foreign substance; similar scar formation can be observed around most other implants, regardless of whether they contain silicone, including hip implants, artificial joints, hydrocephalus shunts, heart valves, and pacemakers. For unknown reasons, in some cases, the scar tissue capsule may become thick and constrict a soft implant. This phenomenon is referred to as capsular contracture. This condition can make the breast feel harder and firmer than desirable, producing a rounded or spherical breast appearance; sometimes it can also cause pain. The severity of this problem varies with each individual. Ideally, the capsular layer surrounding the implant does not contract and affect the shape of the breast. In some women it manifests itself as a slight breast firmness. Mild contracture requires no treatment. Most women find this minimal firmness acceptable and are not motivated to undergo further adjustments of their reconstructed or augmented breasts. In more severe cases of capsular contracture, however, a woman may experience significant discomfort and elect to have an operation to release some or all of the scar tissue (capsulotomy) or to remove it (capsulectomy). During this secondary operation the surgeon may reposition the implant under the pectoralis major muscle if previously placed over the muscle or he may replace it with a textured-surface implant after releasing or removing the capsule. These textured-surface implants appear to have a lower incidence of capsular contracture. It is usually necessary to remove the scar capsule around the smooth implant before replacing it with the textured-surface implant. Patients who continue to experience problems after surgical correction may decide to have their implants removed. After implant removal (explantation), an aesthetic correction such as a breast lift (mastopexy) may be necessary to achieve an optimal breast appearance. A woman should be informed of this possibility. Some women with firm breasts decide to have the implant and scar tissue removed and replaced or covered with fatty and muscle flap tissue from the back, lower abdomen, or buttocks.

Although capsular contracture may be uncomfortable and produce breast distortion and asymmetry, it is not a health hazard. Rarely this contracture may result in the implant being exposed through thin breast skin. It does not, however, threaten a woman's life or health, and most women who experience this problem can have satisfactory surgical correction. With the newer textured breast implants, capsular contracture is estimated to occur in approximately 2% to 4% of cases in some studies and in as many as 4% to 9% of cases in others. These implants have been on the market for 10 years now, and contracture rates with these devices seem to have remained at this level over time.

What can be done to avoid capsular contracture?
Will exercises help?

The incidence of capsular contracture is lower when the implant is placed behind the pectoral muscle. Using implants with a textured covering also seems to reduce the likelihood of capsular contracture; it is thought that the rough surface prevents a smooth, uniform scar from forming and constricting the implant. When smooth-surface implants are used, some surgeons recommend breast massage of the implant throughout the breast pocket in an effort to prevent or reduce the incidence and severity of fibrous capsule formation around the implant. There is no scientific evidence, however, that breast massage is helpful in preventing contracture, and some surgeons have stopped recommending massage to patients with smooth implants. Massage is not necessary for implants with a textured surface.

What are calcium deposits? Can they be mistaken for the calcifications associated with breast cancer?

Sometimes calcium forms in the capsule around the breast implant after it has been implanted for many years. These deposits may increase the hardening; however, they have a characteristic appearance on mammography and can be differentiated from calcifications associated with breast cancer. Breast surgery, including breast reduction, breast lift (mastopexy), and breast reconstruction with a woman's own tissues (autologous), can also cause calcifications visible on mammography.

What effects will breast implant surgery have on breast sensation?

Women having implant surgery for augmentation may experience changes in breast and nipple-areola sensation. Most of these changes are temporary, but in some cases they prove permanent. Women having breast reconstruction with or without implants already have diminished sensation because of the nerves severed during the mastectomy.

Does a woman who has an implant breast reconstruction still need to have mammograms?

Mammograms are usually not necessary after a mastectomy and breast reconstruction. However, if an implant is placed in the opposite breast for symmetry or balance, this breast still needs to be monitored. Women should inform the breast imager that they have a breast implant or expander so that additional displacement views can be taken to help visualize the extent of the breast tissue.

Will breast implants interfere with mammograms?

Both saline-filled and silicone gel–filled implants can pose some imaging problems. Silicone gel–filled implants are opaque to x-rays; saline-filled implants are less so; therefore any breast tissue overlying or underlying the implant may be masked by the implant on the breast films. Women who have implants in place should make sure that they inform the breast imager so that the automatic equipment can be properly adjusted and special displacement views can be taken (in addition to the "standard" or routine mammography compression views) to better visualize the breast tissue. Many physicians recommend that patients with implants should have two additional displacement views. The displacement technique (also known as the Eklund or "pinch" technique) was introduced to allow more breast tissue to be visualized in women with breast implants. With these special views and in the absence of significant capsular contracture, satisfactory breast images can be obtained in most women and their breasts can be effectively monitored for possible breast problems. Both compression and displacement views provide better visualization if the implant has been placed under rather than over the chest wall muscle. The new implant fill materials being studied appear to be more radiolucent and may permit better visualization of breast tissue when an implant is in place.

Should women with implants have more frequent mammograms?

According to Dr. Potchen, "The use of screening mammography in a patient with an implant should be no different than in any other patient. At Michigan State University we currently adhere to the American Cancer Society's guidelines [that recommend yearly mammography for all women 40 years of age and older]. We do not see a need for additional mammographic examinations in individuals who have an implant, and we would not advocate doing mammograms in younger patients." The *FDA Update* of March 1996 further states that "women with breast implants who are in an age group where routine mammograms are recommended should be sure to have these exams at the recommended intervals."

What is the proper way to examine the breasts if a woman has implants?

Like all women, those with breast implants should perform regular breast self-examination (BSE) and have regular physician examinations. These examinations take on added significance for women with breast implants because they can also help to reveal any problems that may develop with their implants.

Can implants slip, shift, or become displaced?

During the initial operation the plastic surgeon places the implant in the best position to provide the desired breast appearance. During the process of healing, with the development of capsular contracture, and over time the implants can shift or become displaced. This can occur because of the pull of gravity on a smooth implant or subsequent to a capsular contracture, which can elevate the implant. This problem occurs less frequently when a textured breast implant has been used because the rough surface usually adheres to the surrounding tissue, thereby minimizing the chance of displacement.

Can the implant be rejected by a woman's body?

"Rejection" means an allergic or immune response that causes the body to literally reject a foreign substance. In this sense implants are not rejected. However, the overlying breast skin may become thinned, infection can develop, or healing may be incomplete, leading to exposure and necessitating removal of the implant. Although these are complications, they are not tantamount to rejection.

Can an implant be removed?

Yes. When an implant is not performing the function for which it was intended, or if the woman feels that she would be better off without the implant, it can be removed. In most cases this is a relatively minor operation, that can often be performed on an outpatient basis. She should ask her plastic surgeon if the capsule should also be removed. The procedure for capsule removal is called capsulectomy. The patient should decide, in consultation with the plastic surgeon, if additional aesthetic corrections will be necessary after removal.

Should women diagnosed with rheumatic diseases have their implants removed?

This is not necessary, according to noted rheumatologists, Drs. John Sergent, Howard Fuchs, and John Johnson. "We do not recommend that women with implants who acquire rheumatic diseases have intact implants removed. It has been recommended for some time that ruptured implants be removed, although this, too, is somewhat controversial if the rupture is contained within the fibrous capsule. If contractures are painful and tender, the decision to remove the implant must be balanced against the expected cosmetic result and the operative risks . . . It is sometimes appropriate to have the implant and associated capsule removed in these patients."

Should women who have polyurethane-coated breast implants consider having them removed?

According to the FDA, "There is insufficient evidence at present to support having polyurethane-coated breast implants surgically removed because of concerns about cancer. The risks of the operation itself to remove or replace the implants are far higher than the risks of keeping the implants."

If a woman needs to have her implants removed because of a problem, or chooses to have them removed because she is concerned about them, will this procedure be reimbursed?

Some insurance carriers will cover implant removal for certain types of problems. The financial arrangements for implant removal should be discussed with your surgeon and your insurance carrier before any decision is made.

What are the manufacturers' replacement policies for saline-filled implants in case of leakage or deflation?

Both McGhan Medical (Inamed) Corporation and Mentor Corporation, the two companies supplying the bulk of saline-filled implants in the United States, offer patients full lifetime replacement in the event of deflation due to loss of shell or valve integrity.

How long do breast implants last?

The silicone breast implant has been available for use in patients since 1964, and many of the original devices are still in place. Just as human and artificial organs can fail and require transplantation, breast implants also may have to be replaced.

No precise figures on the life span of silicone gel–filled or saline-filled implants are available at present. The ongoing clinical studies and product research should help clarify this. It is known that implants can last from a very short time to many years, depending on the surgical technique used, the patient, and her implant. In any case, breast implants should not be considered "lifetime" devices. Women should be followed up by their physicians over the long term so their breasts can be monitored for possible problems as a part of their general health care regimen.

How strong are implants? Will they break on impact? Can they be broken during mammography?

Breast implants are manufactured to specific standards requiring that they resist breast compression as well as multiple and long-term physical stress. These devices, however, are not indestructible. Although the outer shell of the implant is quite sturdy, it can break if subjected to severe physical trauma. A sharp or blunt injury to the chest wall and breast, such as pressure from a seat belt during a car accident, can cause this problem. The envelope can also tear if it is inadvertently cut or nicked by instruments during surgery. Compression views taken during mammography are calibrated to avoid undue pressure that could rupture a breast implant. According to Dr. Potchen, "There is no evidence that compression or displacement mammography has caused implant rupture."

What factors increase the chance that an implant will rupture?

The chance for rupture may increase with the length of time the implant has been in the body and with normal wear and tear. The incidence of rupture is increased when the implant develops folds or rippling on the outer surface. Trauma or injury to the breast also increases the chance of rupture, as may closed capsulotomy (a technique to correct capsular contracture in which strong pressure is applied to the breast to break up the scar tissue around the implant). This technique is less frequently used today and is not recommended by the manufacturers.

What percentage of implants rupture?

Results from recently released clinical studies revealed a low rupture rate of 0.06% for silicone gel–filled implants. Researchers at Mallinckrodt Institute of Radiology and Washington University Medical School in St. Louis have detected a 5% to 6% rate of implant rupture or leakage among the women with implants they studied. Researchers at the Mayo Clinic found a similar rupture incidence of 5.7%. Other reports from Scotland and California revealed even lower rates of rupture.

Earlier model implants, made with thinner envelopes and containing a different gel configuration, are thought to have a higher rate of rupture and leakage. These thin-walled implants, produced in the mid-1970s to the mid-1980s, are no longer being made. Some have suggested that the envelope failure rate seems to increase after 10 years of implantation. Since the mid-1980s a low-bleed implant enve-lope has been used and is more resistant to rupture.

How can a woman tell if she has a ruptured or deflated implant?

Any noticeable change in the shape, size, feel, or comfort of the breast could signal implant rupture. For women with saline-filled implants, this change in breast size and shape is often more noticeable when leakage and absorption of the saltwater solution by the surrounding tissues causes implant deflation. When such symptoms occur, a pa-tient should see her plastic surgeon for evaluation. According to the FDA, "It is possible for a woman to experience rupture of the implant without symptoms, but women should not have routine mammograms (x-rays of the breasts) just to detect these 'silent' ruptures if they are not experiencing any symptoms."

What happens if a saline-filled implant deflates?

There is a possibility of deflation with saline-filled implants if a leak develops in the implant covering and will require possible reoperation with implant replacement. Currently available saline-filled inflatable implants have a relatively low deflation rate. One-year cumulative results from the clinical trials conducted by the two remaining U.S. implant manufacturers reveal deflation rates ranging from 1.7% by one of the companies to 3.7% by the other. A study conducted at the University of Minnesota of 504 patients receiving saline-filled im-plants reported a 5.5% deflation rate. As with silicone gel–filled im-plants, saline-filled implants should not be considered lifetime de-vices.

What happens if a silicone gel–filled implant leaks?

When the cover of a silicone gel–filled implant is pierced or ruptures, the gel usually remains within the fibrous capsule or membrane that develops naturally around the implant and does not travel to other parts of the body. Significant trauma can cause tears in the surround-ing capsule, and the gel can migrate into the breast and possibly be-yond the breast to form lumps (granulomas) nearby. Some of this sili-cone can cause enlarged lymph nodes in the armpit area (lym-phadenopathy). When silicone escapes to other parts of the body, such as the arm or upper abdomen, removal can be difficult. Gel migration outside the capsule rarely occurs, however, and, if it does, the viscosity (or thickness) of the gel seems to reduce its ability to migrate.

What is silicone bleed?

Silicone bleed refers to microscopic amounts of silicone fluid that seep through the implant's envelope. Although most of this is trapped within the implant pocket or the surrounding scar tissue, minute amounts of silicone could possibly migrate through the capsule. The majority of implants manufactured after 1985 have a low-bleed design that reduces leakage.

Can ultrasound, magnetic resonance imaging, or mammography be used to detect implant leakage or rupture?

Ultrasonography is an adjunct to mammography that can be useful in detecting implant rupture. Computed tomography (CT) scans have also been used but require a relatively high dose of radiation compared with mammography. Magnetic resonance imaging (MRI) is not recommended for routine screening, but it is a useful adjunct to mammography for evaluation of implant integrity for possible leakage as well as the actual breast for masses and cancer. Dr. Potchen reports that "MRI is currently the most accurate way of determining whether an implant has ruptured. It is an expensive and perhaps unnecessary approach depending on whether the rupture produces symptoms or is likely to create subsequent problems. It also depends on whether it is a *capsulated* [italics ours] rupture [in which the gel is contained in the capsule that surrounds the implant] or whether silicone has leaked into other tissues. Generally a crude estimate of rupture can be pretty well determined on a mammogram. Even at that, I would not recommend using mammography in patients younger than 30. One advantage of ultrasonography or MRI is that there is no ionizing radiation."

Is there a test to detect silicone in the body or determine whether a woman is sensitive to silicone?

No. According to the FDA, "There is no FDA-approved, standard test to detect silicone in the body. . . . Even if simple techniques for silicone detection were available, they might not be useful in detecting a rupture, because small amounts of silicone ordinarily 'bleed' even from intact implants." Furthermore, since silicone is found in food and many other products, including commonly used medicines and cosmetics, individuals have quantities of silicone in their bodies regardless of whether they have breast implants. Therefore, "the tests would not easily determine whether the silicone came from the implant or another source."

As the FDA has indicated, "Determining that silicon or silicone is present in body fluids does not indicate whether a person is sensitive to these substances or at risk for any specific disease. There is presently no test to determine if a person is sensitive to silicone or silicon."

Do ruptured implants and leakage of silicone gel pose a major health hazard?

Not according to Drs. John E. Woods and Phillip G. Arnold, two plastic surgeons from the Mayo Clinic. In an article in *The Wall Street Journal* they explain that "over the years, we have removed many ruptured implants, not because the patient has complained of any symptoms but simply in the process of releasing capsules or exchanging the implants. We have not seen any serious consequences in patients with ruptured implants. Silicone gel is readily removed from the pocket and has only extremely rarely been associated with postoperative problems. We believe that when ruptures are known to exist, it is appropriate to remove the implants. In most patients, however, the presence of ruptured implants is not detectable, is asymptomatic, and is not likely to cause problems."

A more recent Mayo Clinic study conducted by Drs. John E. Woods and Michael Duffy concluded that their 30-year clinical experience with silicone gel breast implants for augmentation mammaplasty and breast reconstruction "failed to demonstrate that clinically evident adverse health problems are incurred by those women who subsequently experience a silicone gel breast implant failure."

These data do not suggest that women with breast implants are not subject to the usual health problems that affect the population at large. Breast cancer, heart disease, and arthritis, to name a few, are common health problems confronted by all women.

What are the risks if a saline-filled implant ruptures?

Although the safety of saline-filled implants is being evaluated by the FDA, leakage or deflation of these implants results in release of saline solution (saltwater), which is not foreign to the body, thus avoiding some of the concerns associated with silicone gel. (The saltwater is absorbed after it leaks out, resulting in deflation of the implant.) Because saline-filled implants do not contain silicone gel, fewer questions have been raised about their safety; they are still available without restriction for both augmentation and reconstruction. But since both types of implants have an outer silicone elastomer envelope, the long-term safety of which is being studied, the saline-filled implants may not be entirely without risk and are being reviewed by the FDA.

What should be done if an implant ruptures?

If a woman suspects possible implant rupture, she should see her doctor. Many experts recommend that removal of a ruptured implant be considered. Frequently the capsule surrounding the implant or a portion of it may have to be removed at this time. If the implant rupture is confined to the capsule, many women have chosen to avoid an operation, to leave the contained leaking implant in place, and to take a "wait and watch" approach under medical supervision.

What should women with implants do to minimize possible problems?

Women with implants should take the time to inform themselves about their implants. This means finding out specifically what type of implants they have, the date of implantation, the manufacturer, and the model number. They can obtain a copy of the package insert (instructions accompanying the implant and providing information on possible risks and complications for that device model). It is also crucial for all breast cancer patients and for women with implants to practice monthly BSE, to have regular physician examinations, and to report any problems, changes, or concerns to their doctors. They should keep in close contact with their doctors for adequate follow-up. Finally, joining a breast implant registry through the implant manufacturer will help to ensure that women are kept informed about safety issues for these devices. Tracking of breast implants is mandated by the FDA.

Can silicone gel–filled or saline-filled implants cause cancer?

Silicone breast implants have been available for almost 35 years and during that time have been studied extensively by plastic surgeons, implant manufacturers, scientists, and government regulatory agencies such as the FDA. In all of that time no scientific studies have documented an increased risk of breast cancer attributable to breast implants nor is there any evidence that these devices have adversely affected the course of breast cancer when they are used for breast reconstruction. Large population studies from California, Denmark, Sweden, France, and Canada have all indicated that the incidence of breast cancer in women with silicone breast implants is the same or possibly lower than in women who have not had implants. Interestingly, several studies (such as the one conducted in Los Angeles) reported a lower incidence of cancer occurring in women with implants. The FDA's current informed consent document serves to underscore these findings. It states, "There is presently no scientific evidence that links either silicone gel–filled or saline-filled breast implants with cancer."

Is there any scientific evidence to prove that silicone gel–filled implants pose potential dangers to a woman's health?

After studying the information about silicone gel–filled breast implants provided by its consultants, the FDA stated that more data are needed about these devices, but there is no evidence that they cause breast cancer or autoimmune diseases.

What do cancer specialists say about the dangers of breast implants? Is there a risk of cancer from breast implants?

The research from cancer experts and institutions throughout the world seems to indicate a general consensus that breast implants do not increase a woman's risk of developing breast cancer. Studies conducted by researchers from the U.S. National Cancer Institute, the International Epidemiology Institute and the Karolinska Institute in Sweden, the Danish Cancer Registry, the Fred Hutchinson Cancer Research Center, the Institut Gustave Roussy in France, the Alberta Canada Cancer Board, and the U.S. Centers for Disease Control and Prevention, among others, have all found that there was no greater incidence of breast cancer among women with implants than in the general population. Large population studies seem to confirm this finding, such as the one conducted at the University of Southern California School of Medicine, which concluded "that there is no increase in breast cancer incidence following augmentation mammaplasty." Additional studies are under way to study implants and their long-term impact on a woman's health.

What are connective tissue disorders? What symptoms are associated with these diseases?

These are rare disorders such as lupus erythematosus, dermatomyositis, scleroderma, and rheumatoid arthritis in which the body reacts to its own tissue as though it were a foreign material. A combination of symptoms may characterize these disorders, including the generalized symptoms of joint pain and swelling; tight, red, or swollen skin; swollen glands and lymph nodes; extreme fatigue; local symptoms of swelling of the hands and feet; skin rashes; and unusual hair loss.

The FDA advises a woman who experiences these symptoms to "see her regular doctor if the symptoms do not subside, because these complaints could be indicators of a variety of health problems, not just immune-related disorders."

Can implants cause connective tissue or autoimmune disease in healthy women?

There have been allegations that implants can cause or exacerbate immune-related or connective tissue disorders (also referred to as collagen vascular diseases or incorrectly as human adjuvant disease). This possibility has been carefully evaluated by respected immunologists and rheumatologists in numerous national and international scientific studies. The consensus after extensive scientific investigation seems to be that there is no conclusive scientific evidence to indicate that there is an increased incidence of such diseases in patients with breast implants. Although these conditions may exist concurrently, there is no evidence that a silicone implant has caused or contributed to autoimmune disease. Even the FDA's own *Epidemiological Review* published in 1996 concurs that "current research has tended to rule out large increases in risk for connective tissue disease caused by breast implants." Following is an overview of some of the studies that address this question.

Scientific studies conducted at the Mayo Clinic, Harvard Medical School, University of Michigan School of Public Health, Emory University, University of Kansas Arthritis Center, University of Texas M.D. Anderson Cancer Center, University of Washington Fred Hutchinson Cancer Research Center, University of Toronto, University of Maryland, University of Pittsburgh, University of California, San Diego, and Johns Hopkins University Schools of Medicine have revealed no association between silicone gel breast implants and connective tissue disease. The 1996 Women's Health Cohort Study conducted at Brigham & Women's Hospital, Harvard Medical School, evaluated 10,380 women with silicone breast implants and a control group of 384,713 women without implants. After considering all available evidence, this large study concluded that "women with breast implants should be reassured that there is no large risk of connective tissue disease."

In a *New England Journal of Medicine* article published in 1995 Dr. Jorge Sánchez-Guerrero and his colleagues analyzed the data from 14 years of follow-up of a National Institutes of Health (NIH)–funded study from Brigham & Women's Hospital, Harvard Medical School. This study examined the incidence of connective tissue disease and 41 signs, symptoms, or laboratory findings of connective tissue disease among a group of 87,500 registered nurses between the ages of 30 and 55. The authors concluded that "there was no evidence of an association between silicone breast implants and connective-tissue diseases defined according to a variety of standardized criteria or signs and symptoms of these diseases."

International studies have come to the same overall conclusions. Research conducted in Australia, Canada, Denmark, and Sweden also failed to find "a causal relationship between the implantation and the development of connective tissue disease."

An article published in *Arthritis and Rheumatism* summarizes recent research by investigators from Brigham & Women's Hospital, Harvard Medical School, Robert B. Brigham Multipurpose Arthritis Center, Saint Thomas Hospital, and Vanderbilt University School of Medicine. This article reports that the clinical, immunologic, and epidemiologic evidence to date "suggests little or no association between silicone breast implants and CTD [connective tissue disease] or a unique arthralgia/myalgia/fibromyalgia syndrome."

This lack of causal relationship is given additional support and credibility by the American College of Rhematology's Revised Statement on Silicone Breast Implants published in the *Journal of the American Medical Association* in 1996. The College concludes that current large studies "provide compelling evidence that silicone implants expose patients to *no* demonstrable additional risk for connective tissue or rheumatic disease. Anecdotal evidence should no longer be used to support this relationship in the courts or by the FDA."

What advice should rheumatologists and immunologists give to patients contemplating implant surgery?

Dr. John Sergent, a respected rheumatologist, advises informing patients that "a few reports have indicated a relationship between implants and various rheumatic diseases. The number of patients reported is small, and considering the total number of implants, it may not even be a valid observation. If there is a causal relationship, it is clearly a rare event."

Should women diagnosed with connective tissue diseases or autoimmune diseases have reconstruction with breast implants?

These diseases are rare, and scientific studies are under way to define and better understand these conditions. As a precaution, however, if a woman has any of these conditions or has a family history of these conditions, she should probably not have silicone gel–filled or saline-filled implants until the results of current population studies and other information are available. As Dr. John Sergent explains, "My recommendation for patients with scleroderma is to minimize trauma of any kind. That would include all cosmetic surgery, not just implants. Many patients with scleroderma request cosmetic surgery to correct the perioral wrinkles they all have, and I strongly discourage them. Most of them do well with surgery; the skin heals quite well. However, there are some patients who have an exuberant fibrotic reaction. My across-the-board recommendation for patients with scleroderma is that all elective surgery should be avoided—implants or anything else." Women with these problems are also poor candidates for radiation therapy and musculocutaneous flaps.

Can implants cause neurologic disease in healthy women?

According to the American Academy of Neurology, "there really is no evidence from what has been published that breast implants are associated with or cause neurologic disease." Dr. John Ferguson, chairman of the Academy's Therapeutics and Technology Assessment Subcommittee, speculates that the reason many people think breast implants cause health problems is because the FDA took implants off the market in 1992. "That made women think, 'Maybe there's something wrong and maybe this ache or that pain is caused by this device.' I think the women who have complaints are suffering, but I think there's no good evidence from what I can see regarding either autoimmune disease or certainly not in neurologic disease that that's the cause of their problems."

Is it possible to be allergic to silicone implants or to the silicone gel within them?

As mentioned earlier, silicone has been used in medical devices and oral and parenteral medications for over 40 years, and there is no scientific evidence that individuals can develop allergies to these devices. It may be possible, however, to develop antibodies to the silicone. The mere presence of antibodies, however, does not indicate the presence of disease. The body's normal process of dealing with foreign bodies is an immune response with subsequent development of antibodies. Further studies will need to be conducted to determine if there are actually any allergic reactions.

What possible complications can occur with implant surgery?

As with any surgical procedure, there is the potential for complications, including reactions to anesthesia as well as infection, hematoma, bleeding, seroma, and delayed wound healing with possible implant exposure requiring removal.

Are there any recorded deaths from breast implants?

There are no reports in the medical literature of breast implants being responsible for a single death. There is an inherent risk of serious complications and even death from any operation, but this is usually related to the risk of anesthesia for a period of time. This risk is somewhat higher for longer operations, particularly if the operation lasts for more than 4 hours. However, the risk is still considered very small.

How does the incidence of complications from implant surgery compare to the incidence of complications from other common operations such as appendectomies, mastectomies, and hysterectomies?

The rate of complications experienced after breast implantation is comparable to and sometimes lower than the rate of complications from other commonly performed operations. A study by Dr. Sherine Gabriel and colleagues published in the *New England Journal of Medicine* in 1997 examined the rate of local complications requiring reoperation in women with breast implants. The researchers found that approximately 24% of the women studied experienced at least one surgically treated complication over the period of follow-up. According to Dr. Gabriel, "These rates are about the same as the rates reported for breast reconstruction without implants and are comparable to reports from other centers." Patients having breast implant surgery generally have a lower incidence of conditions such as infection, hematoma, pulmonary emboli, and deep vein thrombosis. However, reoperation because of capsular contracture or to achieve a better final breast appearance is necessary in a significant number of cases.

Why don't women just have reconstruction with their own natural tissue from their abdomen, buttock, or back instead of incurring the risks of a foreign material?

Many women want an operation that can be done either as an outpatient procedure or with minimal down time, expense, and inconvenience. For them, implant reconstruction is the best choice because it affords the convenience, short recovery period, and reduced cost they desire. This is also the procedure of choice for a woman who does not want any additional scars, a necessary consequence of most flap procedures. Implant surgery is a good choice for a slender woman who may not have enough fatty tissue for a flap procedure or for a woman with a medical condition that places her at increased risk if she has a more complex operation such as a TRAM (abdominal) flap, latissimus dorsi (back) flap, or a free flap. Furthermore, many surgeons experienced in breast reconstruction techniques with implants and expanders prefer these operations for most patients over the more involved flap procedures.

What are the risks involved with flap surgery? How do these risks compare to those encountered in implant surgery?

The decision to have breast reconstruction with a flap or with a breast implant involves an analysis of the risks and benefits of the two approaches. Flap operations take longer, which means increased risks of major surgical complications such as deep vein thrombosis, pulmonary complications, and fluid retention. The success of flap procedures depends on the blood supply of the flaps; if this is compromised, part or all of the flap can be lost. Fortunately, this is a rare occurrence. The shaping of the flap tissue into a breast form also requires more skill and artistry on the part of the surgeon than that required for placement of a breast implant or expander. The obvious benefit of autologous flap reconstruction is that it creates a lasting, more natural breast symmetry that is usually maintained for a lifetime and uses the woman's own tissues, generally without the need for an implant.

The perioperative risks of implant reconstruction are less serious and pose a lower chance of major complications. The benefits of breast reconstruction with breast implants are also significant for the patient who can have a successful procedure with minimal inconvenience and cost. The drawback of this approach is that a deflation or rupture can occur or a capsular contracture can develop around the breast implant and may require additional procedures in the future. Additionally, implants are not considered lifetime devices and may have to be replaced at some point in the future.

What is the FDA's role in testing and evaluating implants and expanders?

The FDA has been charged with regulating all medical devices since 1976 and is involved in an ongoing evaluation of the safety and efficacy of breast implants. The FDA designates these devices as class III, which means that they must have premarket approval of their safety and efficacy. During the early 1990s the FDA conducted hearings on polyurethane-covered implants and silicone gel–filled implants. Saline-filled implants are currently in the final phases of FDA review. It is anticipated that the final clinical study documentation along with the premarket approval application will be required to be submitted to the FDA on all saline products before the close of 1998.

Why has the FDA evaluated breast implants if they are not dangerous?

The FDA investigation into the safety of silicone breast implants is merely an example of a government agency performing its legally mandated regulatory function. When the FDA was granted authority to regulate medical devices in 1976, 100,000 devices being distributed were required to be registered with the FDA and were permitted to remain on the market pending later review. Breast implants were included on the FDA's list for review, but devices such as heart valves and intrauterine devices (IUDs) were scrutinized first. It took from 1976 until 1988 (when the review process was completed for some of these other devices) before the FDA turned its attention to breast implants and officially placed them into a class III category, a designation assigned to most other permanently implantable medical devices. This classification requires manufacturers to submit comprehensive safety and effectiveness data in order to secure premarket approval. FDA hearings and mandated clinical trials are part of this ongoing review process as silicone gel–filled and saline-filled implants are scrutinized to ensure that they meet certain safety and effectiveness standards.

What is the current ruling concerning silicone gel–filled breast implant availability?

All women desiring silicone gel–filled breast implants are required to enter clinical trials sponsored by the implant manufacturer and approved by the FDA. Any woman who needs an implant for breast reconstruction is permitted access to these trials or studies, including women who have had breast cancer surgery, women with traumatic breast injuries, and women with severe breast or chest wall deformities or asymmetries. Also eligible are women with an existing breast implant that needs to be replaced for medical reasons. Only a very limited number of women are able to receive silicone gel–filled breast implants for reoperative breast augmentation (as a secondary procedure never as a primary procedure), and these women must enroll in strictly controlled clinical studies referred to as adjunct studies. Participants in all of these studies must read and sign a detailed informed consent form, be closely followed by their doctors after their operation, and have periodic checkups for 5 years after implantation. Women in these studies are enrolled in a patient registry established by the manufacturers.

What is a clinical trial?

A clinical trial is basically a controlled study of patients who are receiving a prescribed treatment or combination of treatments. Clinical trials may be used to determine the usefulness of operations, drugs, devices, or treatments as well as their safety and effectiveness and risks and benefits. Each study is designed to answer scientific questions and to find new and better ways to help patients. Clinical trials have long been used in breast cancer research for evaluating new treatments. Often one or more treatments are compared. Currently clinical trials have been designed to study the safety and effectiveness of breast implants. Many of these studies have been completed.

Are women who want these implants for breast augmentation allowed to get them in the United States if they are not participating in the clinical studies?

No. Although silicone gel–filled implants are still manufactured by two companies in the United States, their distribution and use in the United States is restricted to these studies. However, they are widely available in many other countries through their respective National Health Services. In the United States saline implants continue to be widely available for reconstruction and the only alternative for augmentation.

What actions are other countries taking concerning silicone gel–filled breast implants?

Other countries have also investigated the allegations concerning breast implants and their possible link to systemic disease. The British government has concluded that there is "no evidence of any association between breast implants and connective tissue disease and therefore no reason to alter practice or policy in the United Kingdom." The Australian Medical Association issued a statement that said, "Despite legal interest and media publicity, scientific evidence for silicone-associated diseases is lacking." A similar conclusion was reached by a Swedish study of 10,000 women published in the *British Medical Journal* in February 1998. This study found that women who receive breast implants have no increased risk of developing connective tissue disorders.

The European Committee on Quality Assurance and Medical Devices (EQUAM) in Plastic Surgery has issued a consensus declaration stating that "there is conclusive scientific, clinical, immunological, and epidemiological proof that silicone breast implants do not cause identified and recognized autoimmune diseases nor connective tissue diseases. At present there is no scientifically identified 'new disease' caused by silicone implants . . . [and] . . . no such thing as silicone allergy, nor silicone [associated] disease nor intoxication. There is an immune reaction to every foreign body, but this is not identical with immune disease."

Why are women who want implants for augmentation restricted in their access whereas women who want them for reconstruction are not subject to the same restrictions?

The rationale for this distinction seems to go beyond the scientific evidence available. Scientific studies have revealed no evidence to link these devices with cancer or autoimmune conditions. Even so, access to silicone gel–filled breast implants is restricted to all women who need them for breast reconstruction for "compassionate use" but only to a limited number of women desiring them for secondary breast augmentation operations, never for primary augmentation. All women receiving implants must participate in controlled clinical trials. Many physicians and breast cancer patients have questioned the logic of these restrictions. Why are implants not safe for healthy women but okay for women with breast cancer whose immune systems may already be compromised by their bout with cancer?

Why were women with intact older model silicone gel–filled implants told not to have them removed whereas access to the newer models was restricted?

To gather more information on silicone gel–filled breast implants, the FDA requires all women receiving them to enter controlled clinical trials. However, since the scientific information from numerous clinical studies seems to indicate that these devices do not pose a serious health risk (i.e., cause cancer or autoimmune problems), the FDA has advised patients not to have them removed as long as they have not ruptured and continue to give the patient some benefit. The FDA and physicians believe that the risk of an operation, with the attendant anesthetic and operative risks, is far greater than leaving the devices intact. Why have a potentially risky operation to change something that is performing well and is not broken?

Why are silicone implants subject to such stringent regulation when other silicone products are not subject to similar regulations?

Governmental agencies such as the FDA are bound by specific laws and directives in carrying out their regulatory duties. They are also susceptible to political pressures, the press, and individual interest groups. The individuals interested in this product made their positions known and lobbied the FDA to ban silicone gel–filled implants. The agency responded accordingly. Other silicone devices, however, will be reviewed in the future, but lobbying efforts against these silicone products have not been as intense or attracted as much media attention.

What should women who already have silicone gel–filled implants do about their implants?

It is important to bear in mind that most women do not experience serious problems with their implants. Women who are not experiencing any problems with their breast implants should monitor their breasts just as if they did not have implants. This includes careful, monthly BSE, regular physician examination, and breast imaging as recommended. They should also schedule periodical follow-up visits to their plastic surgeon.

What is the status of saline-filled breast implants and tissue expanders?

Saline-filled breast implants, which contain saltwater rather than silicone gel, are currently on the market and available to all patients. In 1993 the FDA directed the two manufacturers of saline-filled implants (Mentor and McGhan Medical) to conduct clinical trials to prove the safety and effectiveness of these products. The company studies focus on frequency of problems such as rupture/deflation, capsular contracture, infection, and short-term complications. Quality-of-life issues are also being examined. Mentor and McGhan Medical have now completed all preclinical testing as well as clinical retrospective and prospective studies. It is anticipated that the FDA will call for all remaining data by the end of 1998.

With silicone gel–filled implants available only to women enrolled in clinical trials, will women who need them for reconstruction be reimbursed as before?

Reimbursement policies of health insurance companies or other health care providers are not determined by government agencies. However, since the legal status of implants used for breast reconstruction has not changed and they are not considered "investigational," there appears to be no reason why reimbursement policies should change. To be certain about payment issues, however, a woman should always check with her insurance company or health care provider before she schedules an operation.

How have the regulations on breast implants affected insurance coverage for women who have already had implant surgery? Is their insurance coverage jeopardized?

This, of course, has been a major concern for individuals with silicone breast implants. Coverage varies with the different companies and group policies and with different health maintenance organizations and managed health care organizations. There is evidence that individual insurance companies with individual policies have sometimes excluded coverage for future breast problems for women with silicone breast implants (even when the problems are not related to their implants). A number of lawsuits have been filed against insurance companies concerning this issue. Now with the accumulating scientific data to support women's claims for coverage, the pendulum seems to be swinging back in their favor.

If a woman wants to have breast implants for reconstruction, what should she do to make sure they are covered by insurance?

Most insurance companies do not cover "cosmetic" surgery; however, they do reimburse breast cancer patients for the costs of breast reconstruction after mastectomy, including the cost of breast implants. Seventeen states now mandate coverage for breast reconstruction, ranging from covering just the mastectomy breast to covering a procedure on the opposite breast (augmentation, reduction, or breast lift) for symmetry or risk prevention (prophylactic mastectomy). Currently, federal legislation is under consideration to mandate breast reconstruction with the option of an opposite breast implant for symmetry. As a precaution, it is best to contact your insurance company before any anticipated operation. Your physician can often provide essential information to give to the insurance company related to the specific medical diagnosis, the specifics of the procedure, and the computer code numbers necessary for predetermination of coverage and an explanation of your benefits under the policy.

In addition, the FDA advises women to get written answers from their insurance company to the following questions:
- Does my policy cover the costs of the implant surgery, the implant, the anesthesia, and other related hospital costs?
- Does it cover treatments for medical problems that may be caused by either the implant or the reconstruction?
- Does it cover removal of the implants if this becomes necessary?

What types of information are we attempting to gather about silicone gel–filled breast implants from the clinical trials and other studies that are being conducted.

The studies are seeking answers to the following questions:
- What is the expected life of implants?
- How often do implants leak or rupture?
- What happens to gel that escapes into the body?
- How do you measure silicone in the body?
- How do you measure sensitivity to silicone?
- How often do women with implants suffer problems?

- Do implants cause or increase the risk of cancer?
- Do implants cause or exacerbate connective tissue disorders?

What types of information are the saline-filled implant clinical trials trying to gather?

The trials are seeking answers to the following questions:
- How often do saline-filled implants leak/deflate?
- What is the incidence of capsular contracture after saline-filled implant surgery?
- How often do infections occur before, during, or after saline-filled implant surgery?
- How often do women with saline-filled implants suffer with short-term complications?
- How does breast implant surgery affect a patient's quality of life?

What is an IDE?

An Investigational Device Exemption (IDE) is a permit that allows a physician to use a device that has not been approved if it is part of a closely controlled clinical study. Participation in an IDE study requires the investigator to supply additional information concerning the safety and effectiveness of the devices. Classification of the study under an IDE ensures that the clinical trials will be structured to gather this information under strictly controlled circumstances. Currently, silicone gel–filled implants used for reconstruction are not included under an IDE, but are monitored under a study referred to as an Adjunct Study.

What does informed consent really mean?

"Informed consent" is a legal term that means that the individual contemplating a certain treatment be fully informed of all of the goals and specifics of the treatment as well as its possible consequences. To be truly "informed" this patient must be provided with this information in verbal and in written form and in terms that are clear and understandable. Risks and benefits of the procedure as well as possible complications and their consequences must be fully described and explained.

What type of informed consent is required for a woman getting silicone gel–filled or saline-filled breast implants?

Informed consent documents for silicone gel–filled and saline-filled implants have been developed by the implant manufacturers in cooperation with the FDA.

What is an implant registry? What is its purpose? Why should a woman participate?

An implant registry is a (FDA-mandated) central computerized data bank established by manufacturers in the implant business. (Former manufacturers do not have registries.) The registry contains pertinent information on patients and their implants. The woman's name, address, and other personal data are kept on file. It also contains information concerning her saline- or silicone-filled breast implant. For the registry to function optimally, this information should be updated periodically. The purpose of the registry is to provide ready access to women who are enrolled so that they can be contacted if there is new information concerning their implants. Information recorded in the registry can also be used to provide data to direct further study of the device. The implant registry is confidential. The FDA is the only group, other than the manufacturers themselves, that has access to this data.

How can a woman find out how to join a registry? Is there a fee?

Each of the two U.S. implant manufacturers still in the implant business provides a registry for women using that company's implants. This type of registry is funded and organized by the manufacturer and there is no fee for participation. A patient can sign up for the prospective (for new patients) or retrospective (for previous patients) registry sponsored by the manufacturer through her doctor. As a member of the registry a patient agrees to inform the registry via change-of-address cards or by calling a toll-free number if her name or address has changed and/or if her implant has been removed or replaced subsequent to implant surgery.

If a woman already has implants, is she still eligible to join an implant registry? Or if she didn't sign up for the manufacturer registry, can she still do so?

Yes. The manufacturers offer both a retrospective registry and a prospective registry. Contact the company that manufactured the implants you have to enroll.

How can a woman find out what type of implants she has?

Women who already have implants can find out what implant was used from their surgeons or from hospital records, if available. Those planning on having implants can ask their surgeons for a photocopy of the "sticker" that identifies the implant by brand name, type, product number, manufacturer, and date of implant. The manufacturers also provide copies of a "Patient Card" that describes the specifics of the device being implanted. Women who had their implant surgery over 15 years ago may have more difficulty locating records of implant specifications for their implants.

How can a woman report problems with her implants?

If a woman develops problems with her implants, she should first contact the doctor who performed her implant surgery. She can also report problems to the company that manufactured the implants. Manufacturers are required by law to report all problems associated with these devices to the FDA. Problems can also be reported directly to the FDA through the MedWatch voluntary reporting system (1-800-FDA-1088), although the FDA recommends physician reporting as the preferred method.

How can a woman sort through the media reports about implants to discover the truth about their safety and efficacy?

That is a difficult question. In our judgment the media is not the place to turn for objective scientific information. Rather, a woman seeking more information about implants or about any medical concern should look to the scientific literature and to respected medical professionals for guidance. She may want to ask her physician to assist her by recommending articles, books, and videotapes on this topic. In addition, the information presented here is culled from the scientific literature and from acknowledged experts. We have included an extensive bibliography to assist the reader in securing more information. The FDA has a toll-free telephone line for consumers (1-800-532-4440); by calling this number women can receive up-to-date, accurate information on silicone breast implants and their regulatory status.

What is the American Cancer Society's position on silicone gel–filled breast implants?

According to the American Cancer Society's position statement, "The American Cancer Society believes that breast implants should continue to be made available as an option in cancer rehabilitation. Any decision regarding breast reconstruction should be discussed by the woman and her physician to determine the individual's benefits and risks. The American Cancer Society supports further research into long-term safety issues related to breast implants."

What are the latest American Medical Association's recommendations concerning silicone breast implants?

In an article published in the *Journal of the American Medical Association* in December 1993 the AMA noted that the FDA hearings were "characterized by excessive emphasis on evidence based on anecdotal opinion rather than . . . scientifically proved data. This imbalance likely facilitated the inappropriate media coverage that produced undue anxiety in women with implants." The AMA recommended (1) establishment of a registry of all patients with breast implants to regularly review and report health outcome data; (2) support for the position that women have the "right to choose silicone gel–filled or saline-filled breast implants for both augmentation and reconstruction after being fully informed about the risks and benefits"; (3) physicians be informed of current scientific data available to address the public anxiety over the safety of breast implants ("an anxiety not warranted based on current scientific evidence"); (4) "continued availability of silicone gel implants for both augmentation and reconstruction provided that there is appropriate data collection and follow-up . . . and that clinical trials as proposed by the FDA do not limit a woman's right to choose"; (5) "the AMA monitor the decision-making process of the FDA on the use of not only silicone gel breast implants, but also all silicone-based devices, with particular attention to use of expert medical judgment and to issues of conflict of interest"; and (6) "the AMA request that specific FDA policies regarding the process of device evaluation be developed and publicized to the medical profession and the public and that the process be sensitive to the emotional impact on the patient."

Why have some manufacturers gotten out of the implant business?

In view of the negative publicity generated by the scrutiny of implants in the national media and the subsequent litigation surrounding this controversy, most implant manufacturers decided that the best business decision was to withdraw from the market in the early 1990s. Many of these were large multinational companies, and for them the breast implant business represented a small contribution to their bottom line.

What companies still sell implants? How have these companies been affected by the FDA rulings? What steps have they taken to ensure the safety of implants?

Currently, there are only two companies in the United States that continue to make breast implants, McGhan Medical and Mentor, and two international companies, PIP and Hutchinson. The two U.S. companies are carefully monitored by the FDA and must meet rigorous criteria for manufacture. They are required to establish registries, participate in ongoing clinical trials, and conduct far-reaching product testing to ensure the continued safety and effectiveness of their products. These companies have completed or are completing numerous tests to evaluate the safety and effectiveness of these devices. They are also involved in research to develop and test new and improved devices. These studies have been ongoing for many years; in addition, new studies are now mandated by the FDA. It is not clear whether PIP and Hutchinson must adhere to similar rigorous standards for their products. They have, however, submitted an application for marketing saline-filled implants in the United States, claiming equivalency to the McGhan Medical and Mentor saline implants.

What part do these companies play in the clinical trials?

The companies play a pivotal role in the clinical trials. In the current studies the companies are required to work with specific doctors and centers around the country who agree to use their implants and to comply with the rules of the study. The companies must provide an FDA-approved protocol to doctors as well as the necessary forms to be completed on each patient. In addition, they must establish and support a patient registry and monitor each participating surgeon for compliance to the protocol. On request from the FDA these companies are also required to collect and organize data on each patient for possible FDA evaluation.

How have FDA regulations affected the price of implants?

The two U.S. companies that continue to manufacture silicone gel–filled breast implants must contend with a smaller market, decreased consumer demand, higher costs associated with implementing FDA regulations and financing registries, the expense of clinical trials and studies, and substantial legal costs. These additional financial and workload burdens have understandably increased their cost of doing business. To remain in business they must pass this cost on to the consumer. Consequently, the cost of breast implants has risen approximately 300% and most likely will continue to rise as new technologies are introduced.

Will implant manufacturers discontinue manufacturing silicone gel? What alternate fillings are being suggested?

Both remaining U.S. manufacturers are committed to the silicone gel market. Their clinical studies will be presented to the FDA for approval. Various new substances that promise to be radiolucent and easily absorbed by the body are under development. It is hoped that these fillings can be evaluated under the current clinical trials so that they can receive FDA approval and be used as alternative fills.

What role have the manufacturers played in the silicone implant debate?

The manufacturers have played a key role in the breast implant debate, and these companies have been the subject of intense scrutiny and publicity. Some plastic surgeons believe that they relied too heavily on the companies for supportive data, and now question the accuracy of some of the information that they received. All parties acknowledge that over the years these companies have invested enormous resources in developing, testing, and improving their products and in conducting ongoing research. Critics think that the companies were initially lax in conducting the specific studies needed to assess the long-term efficacy and safety of these devices and to meet FDA standards for premarket approval. Perhaps they should have taken the lead in coordinating follow-up with plastic surgeons to assess the rate and severity of complications. If they had established a better dialogue with the FDA, misunderstandings may have been avoided. However, some of the responsibility clearly lies with the FDA. It was not until 1991 that these companies were given any formal guidance as to the specific testing that the FDA wanted performed. The companies therefore could not be certain what the FDA wanted until just before the results of their product research were to be submitted for review. If this guidance had been provided earlier, with better communication on both sides, the manufacturers' dollars and research efforts could have been directed with those goals in mind, providing ready answers to questions about safety and efficacy and avoiding much of the controversy that has surrounded these devices.

Most would agree, including the independent investigators, that there were no deliberate cover-ups or wrongdoing. None of the information that has been disclosed indicates that these mistakes resulted in increased risk to the health and safety of women with implants. Furthermore, once the FDA informed the manufacturers of what testing requirements they were expected to meet, these companies cooperated with the FDA to provide full disclosure, to set up the additional studies that the FDA requested, and to produce the information that the FDA demanded. It is unfortunate that this information was not requested and gathered years earlier so that it would have been available to answer the FDA's queries and to prevent the concerns and fears that resulted.

The manufacturers are also continuing to fund research to address potential complications and to investigate whether breast implants are associated with systemic disease.

What role have lawyers played in the silicone implant debate?

Reports in the press and media have pointed out the close relationship of the plaintiff's bar and the consumer advocacy groups that have been vocal in pressing the FDA to ban breast implants. Prior to the escalation of the breast implant debate, lawyers' groups set up special committees and organizations to solicit women as potential plaintiffs in lawsuits against the implant companies. The plaintiff lawyers' trade group, the Association of Trial Lawyers of America, set up a special Breast Implant Litigation Group. Numerous ads were placed in newspapers and on television encouraging women to contact these attorneys to report problems with implants.

The plaintiff's bar requires continuous product liability activity to thrive. Contingency-fee lawyers get approximately one third or more of the money awarded in such cases. The banning of these implants would provide them with a virtual gold mine in potential lawsuits to be filed against the implant manufacturers. As *The Wall Street Journal* reports, "The business of the contingency-fee lawyers . . . is speculating in litigation, hoping to hit deep pockets with big awards, of which they pocket a third or more." Numerous lawsuits have been filed against implant companies and individual physicians. And, as reported in the *Boston Globe* in a story headline that read "Lawyers Fight Over Limits of Implant Trials," these lawyers were also locked in battle with each other over the perceived rewards.

Have the courts decided on the safety of silicone breast implants?

Early in the implant debate, a panel of federal judges consolidated supervision of the silicone implant cases nationwide and assigned it to U.S. District Judge Sam C. Pointer, Jr., in federal court in Birmingham,

Alabama. Judge Pointer has played a major role in negotiating the various settlements and in adjudicating this issue and assessing the scientific evidence presented in these cases.

What steps have been taken by judges to ensure that decisions about implant safety are based on reliable scientific evidence?

Judge Pointer has convened a scientific panel of four doctors (a rheumatologist, a toxicologist, an immunologist, and an epidemiologist) to hear scholarly presentations from scientists on both sides of this issue to evaluate current evidence of whether silicone may cause human immune system illnesses. Extensive documents, including studies and reports, have been submitted to the panel for their review and consideration. The establishment of a national science panel has been widely applauded by the medical community and the manufacturers who have pushed to have decisions on implant safety based on sound scientific evidence from well-defined studies and not on what has widely been termed "junk science" whereby so-called hired experts provide anecdotal (personal) stories and opinions that are not verifiable.

Another landmark judicial decision in support of sound science in the courtroom was made by Judge Robert E. Jones, of the U.S. District Court for the District of Oregon on December 27, 1996. Judge Jones ruled that plaintiff's evidence supporting a link between silicone breast implants and serious systemic disease did not meet the standard for scientific proof and therefore was inadmissible in court and should not be presented to juries under the Supreme Court's test in *Daubert v. Merrill Dow Pharmaceuticals, Inc.* (The Supreme Court instructed trial courts to make better use of their gatekeeping authority to keep unproved scientific evidence out of the courtroom and to aggressively screen out ill-founded or speculative theories.)

How have recent court decisions been affected by reliance on the Daubert standards for evaluating scientific evidence in silicone implant cases?

Rulings from judges are beginning to match the judgments of the scientific community finding insufficient evidence to support claims that silicone implants cause disease. For example, in February 1997, in *Pick v. American Medical Systems, Inc.,* Judge Ginger Berrigan of the U.S. District Court for the Eastern District of Louisiana issued a Daubert decision granting a summary judgment excluding the testimony of 13 plaintiffs' disease causation experts. In *Kelly v. American*

Heyer-Schulte in January 1997, Judge Edward Prado of the U.S. District Court for the Western District of Texas ruled in favor of Baxter Healthcare Corporation in a case in which the plaintiff claimed that silicone implants caused her systemic disease. Citing the Daubert case, Judge Prado excluded testimony from the plaintiffs' disease causation experts.

What is the current status of implant settlement talks? Have any settlements been reached? What are the provisions of these settlements?

The breast implant controversy that arose in 1992 resulted in a virtual onslaught of litigation and court cases. Plaintiffs' attorneys sought to recover damages from the manufacturers for possible systemic diseases and other local complications that their clients claimed had been caused by silicone gel implants. To stem the flood of litigation and resolve this issue, the manufacturers began discussing plans for a settlement.

In 1993 a proposed settlement for Mentor was approved by the court. It established a $24 million fund to cover patients who received Mentor silicone gel–filled or saline-filled implants between April 1, 1984, and June 1, 1993. This settlement has proceeded as planned, and Mentor payments or dispersements have already been made to claimants. Three types of payments were provided with this settlement. They included payments for patients who (1) only had Mentor implants, (2) had Mentor or Bioplasty implants, and (3) had Mentor implants and implants from one other manufacturer.

In 1994 a number of the other implant manufacturers proposed a "no liability" $4.25 billion Global Class Settlement (in response to a class action lawsuit filed in federal district court in Birmingham, Alabama). The settlement granted compensation to women who claimed that breast implants manufactured by any of these companies caused a variety of diseases and afflictions. The Global Settlement Plan was dissolved after Dow Corning Corporation filed for Chapter 11 bankruptcy protection. Subsequently, a Revised Settlement Program, which provides for a smaller class action settlement, was proposed.

What are the terms of the Revised Settlement Program and who does it cover?

The Revised Settlement Program involves Baxter HealthCare, Bristol-Meyers Squibb, 3M (Minnesota Mining and Manufacturing), and

McGhan Medical Corporation. The court approved this plan in 1995. The Revised Settlement Program provides a fund to compensate women who have health complaints associated with breast implants manufactured by these companies. It is divided into two categories: Current Claimants and Other Registrants who satisfy certain disease and severity criteria. The benefits for Current Claimants range from $10,000 to $50,000. The benefits for Other Registrants range from a minimum of $75,000 to a maximum of $250,000, depending on the disease and severity level.

The Revised Settlement Program covers U.S. women with silicone breast implants, saline-filled breast implants, and breast implants with polyurethane coverings manufactured by one of the participating companies. Current and future claims for a 15-year period will be reimbursed for medical diagnosis and evaluation, removal of breast implants and implant rupture, as well as specific diseases such as immune system, rheumatologic, or neurologic disorders. Women who wanted to preserve their right to file a claim during the 15-year time period were required to register a claim with the court. The opt-out period has now expired for most registrants. This settlement has proceeded as planned and payments or dispersements are being made to claimants.

The Dow Corning Corporation Chapter 11 bankruptcy is a completely independent court proceeding from the Revised Settlement Program. Women who became members of the class in the Revised Settlement Program must sign up separately by filing a bankruptcy Proof of Claim Form with the Bankruptcy Docketing Agent if they also wish to assert claims against Dow Corning Corporation.

How were women notified about the Revised Settlement Program?

Women were notified of settlement details and requirements for participation through worldwide advertisements and announcements. Fairness hearings were also held by Judge Sam C. Pointer. A toll-free hotline number (1-800-887-6828) was established to provide information on the Revised Settlement Plan. Information could also be obtained on the Internet on Judge Pointer's home page.

Women did not need an attorney to participate in the settlement. They could register with the court if they had no current problem and had recourse for the next 15 years should problems develop. They also did not need to prove that their illness was caused by breast implants to become part of the settlement. They only had to meet the court's criteria for the various funds. This latter point was particularly important in light of the results of numerous studies that are now available and show no link between breast implants and disease.

Why did Dow Corning declare bankruptcy? What impact will this have on claims that have been filed against the company?

Dow Corning filed for protection under Chapter 11 of the U.S. Bankruptcy Code on May 15, 1995, due to extensive litigation and lack of support from their insurers. The company had been a named defendant in an extensive class action lawsuit against several silicone breast implant manufacturers in which a tentative Global Settlement was reached. However, thousands of implant recipients opted out of the Global Settlement and filed individual lawsuits against Dow Corning. By mid-1995 the company was facing dozens of trials each month in locations throughout the United States involving hundreds of plaintiffs. The company then filed for Chapter 11 bankruptcy protection to reorganize its affairs under the supervision of the Bankruptcy Court.

Filing for bankruptcy was not an admission of the validity of the claims filed against the company, but rather a process by which such claims could be resolved. According to Richard Hazleton, Chairman and CEO of Dow Corning, "the time had come to resolve this situation in everyone's best interest."

Where does Dow Corning's Chapter 11 case currently stand?

In February 1998 Dow Corning filed an amended Plan of Reorganization to settle breast implant claims. The Bankruptcy Court must first approve the documents related to this proposed plan before Dow Corning can send it out to claimants for a vote. In addition, the Tort Committee, composed primarily of lawyers representing women with breast implant claims, has filed a motion to withdraw Dow Corning's exclusive right to send its plan out for a vote. A hearing on these matters is scheduled for April 1998.

When will women be able to vote on a plan?

Voting on a plan is a court-supervised process. If the court approves sending a plan out for a vote in the spring of 1998, claimants could begin receiving information and a ballot in the summer of 1998. Whenever the voting period begins, women will have several weeks to make a decision and will not need to take any action until they fully understand the plan. Anyone who has filed a claim in Dow Corning's case will receive the required information for voting through the mail.

What are the proposed terms of Dow Corning's most recent plan?

Dow Corning's $4.4 billion Revised Settlement Plan targets $3 billion primarily for resolving breast implant claims. The balance of those funds would satisfy commercial claims. The new plan offers women more than 15 different settlement choices with payments ranging from $1000 to $200,000—or more for women who have uninsured medical bills that exceed their settlement payments. The plan is designed to provide a range of choices so that women can select the best option to meet their individual circumstances. Settlement options are available over the 16 years of the plan so that women who may want to file claims in the future have a reasonable safety net.

How does Dow Corning's plan address rupture claims or explantation surgery?

The plan offers expanded payments for women whose implants were found ruptured following removal surgery. Payments for those claims range from $15,000 to $50,000, depending on the severity of the rupture. Women who may want to have their implants removed in the future would have access to a Medical Procedures Program to cover the costs related to removal and reconstruction (if that is their choice) as well as a $1000 payment to cover personal expenses.

How does Dow Corning's plan address medical conditions?

Dow Corning's plan offers payments for medical conditions or symptoms ranging from $5000 to $200,000, depending on the level of severity and disability. Women who have uninsured medical bills that exceed their settlement can also file for additional payments.

What if a woman doesn't have anything wrong now, but she filed a claim in case her condition changes. How does Dow Corning's plan address claims filed in the future?

Dow Corning's plan provides a 16-year period to file claims. Women can file a claim for a qualified medical condition at any time during that period and be eligible for the same payments as women who file claims immediately. Furthermore, if a woman settles a claim for a medical condition with a payment of less than $50,000 and her condition later changes, she can refile a claim for an additional payment up to $50,000. Women also will have access to a Medical Procedures Program that will operate over the 16-year period. This program covers the costs involved with removing an implant and reconstruction if a woman so chooses.

Does the manufacturer's willingness to settle suggest that silicone breast implants are linked to serious disease?

The willingness of the manufacturers "to settle" does not signify that silicone implants are harmful. In fact, a growing number of scientific studies conducted by independent researchers at prestigious institutions such as the Mayo Clinic, Johns Hopkins Medical School, and the University of Texas M.D. Anderson Cancer Center have shown that women with implants have no greater incidence of systemic disease than women without implants and that there is no link with cancer. These settlements have been proposed by the manufacturers to provide reasonable and timely options for women to resolve their claims and as a more sensible financial alternative than litigating each case independently, which would likely result in bankruptcy for some companies as it has for Dow Corning. It is estimated that the manufacturers were paying in excess of $1 million per litigated case in legal fees with none of this money going to patients. A settlement seemed the logical solution for all involved. The companies believe that protracted litigation will not be in the best interests of women or the manufacturers. The goal is to resolve this controversy, address claims, and return to normal business operations.

Why did so many different consumer groups present themselves as spokesmen for women in the implant debate? Which groups truly represent women's interests?

It is often difficult to distinguish among the many consumer and support groups that speak for women's interests. Many women have complained that these groups misrepresent themselves as impartial support groups for women seeking information, whereas in reality they represent a specific bias. Women have complained that these groups do not provide them the balanced information they desire.

Potential conflict-of-interest allegations raised against the most vocal of these consumer groups, the Public Citizen Health Research Group, focused on the group's possible ties to the American Trial Lawyers Association. Some have suggested that this group can profit from the banning of these devices and that this organization is indebted to plaintiffs' attorneys for some of its funding. In an article in *Forbes*, several plaintiffs' attorneys were quoted as openly admitting to supporting the organization "overtly, covertly, in every possible way." Additionally, *The Wall Street Journal* reported that "the Public Citizen Health Research Group has prepared how-to kits on suing implant manufacturers; plaintiffs' lawyers pay the group $750 per kit."

To determine if a group will provide the unbiased scientific information you seek we suggest that you start by asking your physician about the names of groups that may be helpful. Many hospitals have support groups set up to aid breast cancer patients and their families. You might also check with the local chapter of the American Cancer Society for names of groups in your area. In addition, Y-ME, the largest national support organization for breast cancer patients, and NABCO, the National Association of Breast Cancer Organizations, are excellent, reliable sources of balanced information.

What experts should a woman consult about the advisability of breast implants for breast reconstruction or cosmetic breast surgery?

The woman considering breast surgery that involves breast implants should obtain detailed information about these devices before deciding if they are for her. Plastic surgeons are well informed about breast implants and can give detailed information. If questions remain, she should consult with her individual physician or surgeon. Information is also available from the FDA, the manufacturers, the American Society of Plastic and Reconstructive Surgeons (1-800-636-0635), and Internet sites of respected medical groups and associations.

PUTTING THE ISSUE INTO PERSPECTIVE

Now that the media hype has subsided and the scientific studies have been completed, what does it all mean? What are the ramifications for women desiring implant surgery? Are the dangers real or have they been distorted? What is the impact on women, their choices, their health care, and ultimately their peace of mind?

Evaluating the Risks

The growing preponderance of available scientific evidence suggests and many credible experts agree that there are no lurking dangers that should unduly alarm us. Most women are not in any serious danger from silicone gel–filled or saline-filled implants or expanders. As the FDA itself has concluded, "These devices do not present a health hazard." As is true of all surgical procedures and all implantable devices, benefits must be weighed against associated problems, risks, and complications, and women need to be alert to these dangers and fully informed about them.

Most women, however, do not experience serious complications from breast implants. Ongoing surveys of women who have had breast implant surgery continue to indicate a high satisfaction level. When queried, most women indicate that they would choose to have implant surgery again. These devices have been used for almost 35 years, and if they had been linked to serious, debilitating health problems, surely we would have heard about it by now, not only in association with implants but in connection with the numerous devices, medications, and products that contain silicone and are widely ingested, injected, or implanted. Silicone is a commonly used material; there are few people in our society who do not have minute quantities of silicone in their bodies as a result of normal activities of daily life.

Defining the Problems: The Scientific Process

What of the women who have experienced serious health problems after implant surgery? Their concerns and anguish are not to be minimized, but the source of their problems needs to be scrutinized more closely. Are these conditions a result of the operation itself, are they associated with the implants, or are they coincidental? This investigation should be conducted not by lawyers in a courtroom, not by expert witnesses receiving payment for their testimony, not by the media in the headlines and on the talk shows, not by self-proclaimed consumer groups receiving funding from malpractice attorneys, but by skilled scientists with expertise in this area who have no special interests beyond the quest for answers to these women's problems. We need to examine the source of these problems to determine why they occurred and how they can be prevented or alleviated. It is a disservice to women to attribute particular symptoms to implants when in fact these problems may have another cause that could be effectively treated if correctly diagnosed.

Peer review and randomized studies are the raw materials that have long supported the scientific process. These well-respected scientific methods were largely ignored as the FDA hearings became politicized and sensationalized. Recent judicial decisions, however, have served to reverse the trend to junk science in the courtroom and to confirm the need for valid scientific evidence as a basis for judicial decision making. It is time to redirect our efforts in the interest of women and of scientific progress.

FDA Ruling: Positives and Negatives

Although some may disagree with the FDA handling of the breast implant evaluation process and with the specifics of its ruling, most would concur that the goal of obtaining reliable scientific information to answer the question of implant safety and effectiveness is admirable and worth pursuing. The FDA sought more information about possible health problems related to the use of these devices. The ruling called for additional detailed scientific studies while allowing the use of silicone gel–filled breast implants under certain limited provisions. Similar studies were also required for saline-filled breast implants; the results of these studies are now becoming available.

These clinical trials have provided positive benefits. They ensure comprehensive informed consent and follow-up for all women having silicone gel–filled implants for breast surgery as well as for those having saline-filled implants. They are designed to provide a means for discovering the true incidence of problems experienced by women who have had these devices implanted, such as the rate of rupture, deflation, infection, and contracture. Additionally, they can look for possible links between these devices and other health conditions.

In the United States access to the clinical trials and to silicone gel–filled implants is available to all women seeking breast reconstruction after mastectomy or for other breast deformities but is strictly limited to a small number of women requesting reoperative breast augmentation. The distinction between breast reconstruction patients and augmentation patients seems to interject a moral judgment in what should be a scientific investigation. The trials should study the safety of these devices, not whether some women have a "better" or more "pressing" need for them. Access to saline-filled implants is not similarly restricted to a specific group of patients; they are used for both augmentation and reconstructive purposes.

Impact of Breast Implant Controversy on the Doctor-Patient Relationship

The implant controversy called into question the competence and motives of medical professionals. They became targets of much media criticism; malpractice attorneys sought to isolate them, along with the implant manufacturers, as villains in the implant debate, even though implants, the object of these attacks, were satisfactory to the vast majority of patients and had never been proved unsafe. As a result, women's confidence in their doctors (particularly in plastic surgeons since they perform implant surgery) was eroded. This was unfortunate. The ties that bind patients to their doctors are crucial to patient well-being. Women facing breast cancer need to have a positive attitude and faith that their doctors will recommend the best treatment and provide the best care possible. They need to know that their doctors are on their team and are committed to helping them.

Few will benefit from this erosion of confidence, certainly not women or the doctors who care for them. If plastic surgeons erred in this scenario, it was by acts of omission, not acts of commission. They could have taken the lead years earlier in establishing registries for better patient follow-up and designing and implementing clinical and research studies on the long-term safety and viability of these devices. They could have worked with the manufacturers to provide a comprehensive, understandable informed consent document to be used for all patients contemplating implant surgery. Most likely they were lulled into complacency by the high level of patient satisfaction and low incidence of complications that they saw after implant surgery. If these measures had been taken, the hysteria generated over the safety of breast implants may have been averted. The much-needed supporting studies and data would have been available to address questions raised.

The female half of this writing team has spent the past 21 years observing and working with doctors and has generally been impressed with their genuine desire to provide optimal health care. Some are indeed more skilled than others, some are better communicators than others, and some are more devoted to their patients than others, but this is true of all people, all professionals. The ongoing FDA scrutiny of breast implants should not reflect on the motives of all caregivers who used them, often in response to patient desires. This is not to excuse those individuals who may not have acted in the best interest of their patients, particularly those physicians who were not qualified to perform implant surgery. But a few bad actors should not cast doubt on the total performance. It would be unfortunate if the implant debate served to permanently undermine the doctor-patient relationship. When a woman is diagnosed with breast cancer, she needs to have confidence that her doctors will help her survive and overcome this life-threatening disease.

Impact of Breast Implant Controversy on Women

For breast cancer patients who have had reconstruction with implants, the breast implant controversy was anxiety provoking. Some of these women were led to believe that their reconstructive implants posed as serious a threat as the cancer they survived. Some were made to feel that they had "time bombs" implanted in their breasts; others were hounded by guilt for having wanted to restore their missing breasts. An atmosphere of fear was generated in the name of women, but not in their interest.

The restriction of silicone gel–filled breast implants primarily to breast reconstruction patients has unfairly penalized and stigmatized women who seek to enhance their self-image. Furthermore, it served to negate some of the positive psychological benefits of reconstructive surgery, sending a message to breast cancer patients that implants are not safe for healthy women. For many breast cancer patients, the doctor's recommendation for breast reconstruction is a sign that their prognosis is good and he considers them candidates for the same type of breast surgery as normal, healthy women. Now this positive reinforcement has been blunted. This may not have been the message that the FDA intended to send, but it was the message that the process delivered.

Healthy women have also been affected by this decision. Many cancer experts believe that breast reconstruction is a lifesaving option for many women who would delay seeking care for breast problems for fear of breast loss. (Implant reconstruction represents the least expensive, least complicated, least time consuming, and therefore one of the most frequently selected methods of breast restoration.) If women are aware that such rehabilitation is available, the hope is that they will be encouraged to practice BSE, to get regular physical examinations, and to go for regular mammograms. Thus, if a cancer is found, it will be in an earlier, more curable stage. Unfortunately, many women will now continue to regard implants, all implants, as hazardous despite the results of subsequent studies. Our surveys and interviews with women over the past 15 years confirm that some will choose to avoid or delay seeking treatment for a breast lump because of their overwhelming fear of breast mutilation. According to some reports, only 50% of the women who discover a breast lump see a doctor within 1 month, and 20% wait a year or more before seeing a physician. Delay in seeking treatment could be a serious blow to the progress that has been made in the early detection of breast cancer.

A Woman's Decision

Women's rights continue to be assailed from many quarters. The FDA in its ruling regarding silicone gel breast implants limited a woman's right to make an informed decision in consultation with her doctor about her own health care. This is a personal decision, but the FDA inserted itself between a woman and her doctor. As Peter Huber, author of *Galileo's Revenge: Junk Science in the Courtroom*, aptly points out in an article in *Forbes*, "If the state can regulate whether or not a woman can put a bag of silicone into her chest, it obviously can also regulate whether she can put an aspirator into her uterus or a contraceptive pill into her mouth. . . . Given all the recent publicity, no one can even plausibly claim that a woman who now opts in favor of a silicone implant has not been fully informed of the risks. If anything, she has been overinformed. The choice should now be hers. . . . When you compromise on the principle of personal autonomy—of freedom of individual choice—you are soon left with all compromise and no principle. . . . A breast implant, safe or dangerous, intact or ruptured, is still just a bag of plastic. When a woman stands in her doctor's office discussing a breast implant, there's only one body and one life involved: her own."

*   *   *

The decision of the FDA and the sensational stories of the media that surfaced in 1992 portrayed women as pawns and second-class citizens. According to Peter Huber, the entire debate "revolved around a vision of vain, foolish, helpless women—women at the mercy of manipulative doctors and conspiring chemical companies, women more like children than adults, women incapable of making intelligent, individual choices for themselves." Those of us who know and work with women with breast cancer know that this is not the case. Women can only gain control over this devastating disease if they have the necessary information and knowledge, and most women who investigate breast cancer treatment and breast reconstruction do so with great intelligence and diligence.

 *Getting the Priorities Straight*

Breast cancer is an overriding threat for all women. It is the most common malignancy in American women, with approximately 180,000 new cases diagnosed each year. It is also the second most common cause of cancer death in women; this year alone over 45,000 women will die from this disease. It seems somehow frivolous for the media and the government to focus so much time and money on breast implants when the real culprit remains virtually ignored.

The breast implant debate has now subsided, the scientific evidence is in, and women can now feel relieved and reassured that their fears about possible serious health concerns tied to breast implants have proved unfounded. As time passes, many women reading this material will be unaware of the controversy that raged and will not be faced with the same issues and concerns. Breast implants are not perfect, but they are not the public enemy that they have been portrayed, and they probably did not warrant all of the attention that they received. The positive psychological, aesthetic, and physical benefits they confer have been all but overlooked in a media blitz of unparalleled proportions. If these devices had not been implanted in women's breasts but rather in some other area of the body, they probably would not have received such widespread attention.

This discussion has attempted to examine the issues and controversies surrounding silicone gel and saline implants based on logic and scientific evidence. We now know a lot more about these devices, and the good news is that they do not pose any serious threat to a woman's health. The scientific evidence is convincing and, hopefully, the media that made the implant controversy front-page news can now give science its fair share of coverage. We hope that this discussion will provide women with the information they need to alleviate some of the anxiety that has been generated and allow them to direct their attention to a far more ominous threat that confronts them. Breast cancer is the enemy, and women need to be fully empowered to face this serious challenge.

BIBLIOGRAPHY

American Cancer Society Documents 002197 & 003068 (1-800-ACS-2345).

American College of Rheumatology Statement on Silicone Breast Implants. October 1995.

The American disease [editorial]. The Wall Street Journal, January 20, 1992.

American Society of Clinical Oncology. American Society of Clinical Oncology and cancer patients seek to ease FDA restrictions on silicone breast implants [press release]. September 19, 1996.

Angell M. Breast implants—Protection or paternalism? N Engl J Med 326:1695, 1992.

Angell M. Do breast implants cause systemic disease? Science in the courtroom. N Engl J Med 330:1748, 1994.

Angell M. Science on Trial: The Clash of Medical Evidence and the Law in the Breast Implant Case. New York: W.W. Norton & Company, 1996.

Angell M. Shattuck Lecture—Evaluating the health risks of breast implants: The interplay of medical science, the law, and public opinion. N Engl J Med 334:1513, 1996.

Berket H, Birdsell DC, Jenkins H. Breast augmentation: A risk factor for breast cancer? N Engl J Med 326:1649, 1992.

Birdsell DC, Jenkins H, Berket H. Breast cancer diagnosis and survival in women with and without breast implants. Plast Reconstr Surg 92:795, 1993.

Breast Implants—An Information Update. Rockville, Md.: U.S. Food and Drug Administration, Department of Health & Human Services, July, 1997.

The breast implant tragedy. Review & outlook. The Wall Street Journal, May 19, 1995.

Brinton LA, Malone KE, Coates RJ, et al. Breast implants and subsequent breast cancer risk. Am J Epidemiol 141:S85, 1995.

Brinton LA, Malone KE, Coates RJ, et al. Breast enlargement and reduction: Results from a breast cancer case-control study. Plast Reconstr Surg 97:269, 1996.

Brody GS, Conway DP, Deapen DM, et al. Consensus statement on the relationship of breast implants to connective-tissue disorders. Plast Reconstr Surg 90:1102, 1992.

Brown SL, Silverman BG, Berg WA. Rupture of silicone-gel breast implants: Causes, sequelae and diagnosis. Lancet 350:1531, 1997.

Bruning N. Breast Implants: Everything You Need to Know. Alamed, Calif.: Hunter House, 1992.

Bryant H, Brasher PMA, van de Sande JG, Turc JM (Alberta Cancer Board). Review of methods in breast augmentation: A risk factor for breast cancer? N Engl J Med 330:293, 1994.

Burns CJ, Liang TJ, Gillespie BW, et al. The epidemiology of scleroderma among women: Assessment of risk from exposure to silicone and silica. J Rheumatol 23:1904, 1996.

Burton TMA. Harvard study finds no major link between implants and immune illnesses. The Wall Street Journal, June 22, 1995.

Burton TMA, Woo J. Lawyers contest implant class action. The Wall Street Journal, March 16, 1992.

Chandler PJ Jr. An outcome analysis of 100 women after explanation of silicone gel breast implants and connective tissue disease and other rheumatic conditions following breast implants in Denmark. Ann Plast Surg 40:103, 1998.

Citizen Petition to FDA requesting that FDA "ease restrictions on availability of silicone gel breast implants for use in women with breast cancer, at high risk for the disease or who have special medical needs." Petition signed by the American Cancer Society, American Society of Clinical Oncology, Cancer Care, Inc., Candlelighters Childhood Cancer Foundation, National Coalition for Cancer Survivorship, Society of Surgical Oncology, US TOO International, Y-ME National Breast Cancer Organization, September 19, 1996.

Cook RR, Delongchamp RR, Woodbury M, et al. The prevalence of women with breast implants in the United States—1989. J Clin Epidemiol 48:519, 1995.

Council on Scientific Affairs, American Medical Association. Silicone gel breast implants. JAMA 270:2602, 1993.

Deapen DM, Bernstein L, Brody GS. Are breast implants anticarcinogenic? A 14-year follow-up of the Los Angeles study. Plast Reconstr Surg 99:1346, 1997.

Deapen DM, Brody GS. Augmentation mammoplasty and breast cancer: A five-year update of the Los Angeles study. J Clin Epidemiol 48:551, 1995.

Deapen DM, Pike MC, Casagrand JT, et al. The relationship between breast cancer and augmentation mammoplasty: An epidemiologic study. Plast Reconstr Surg 77:361, 1986.

Destouet JM, Monsees BS, Oser RF, et al. Screening mammography in 350 women with breast implants: Prevalence and findings of implant complications. AJR 159:973, 1992.

Duffy MJ, Woods JE. Health risks of failed silicone gel breast implants: A 30-year clinical experience. Plast Reconstr Surg 94:295, 1994.

Edworthy SM, Martin L, Barr SG, et al. A clinical study of the relationship between silicone breast implants and connective tissue disease. J Rheumatol 25:254, 1998.

Elkund GW, Busby RC, Miller SH, et al. Improved imaging of the augmented breast. AJR 151:469, 1988.

Englert HJ, Brooks P. Scleroderma and augmentation mammoplasty—A causal relationship? Aust N Z J Med 26:349, 1996.

Englert HJ, Morris D, March L. Scleroderma and silicone gel breast prostheses—The Sydney study revisited. Aust N Z J Med 26:349, 1996.

FDA Talk Paper. TDA and Polyurethane Breast Implants. June 28, 1995.

Feder BJ. A war baby, versatile silicone now shows up everywhere. The New York Times, December 29, 1991.

Fee-Fulkerson K, Conway MR, Winer EP, et al. Factors contributing to patient satisfaction with breast reconstruction using silicone gel implants. Plast Reconstr Surg 97:1420, 1996.

Ferguson JH. Silicone breast implants and neurologic disorders—Report of the practice committee of the American Academy of Neurology. Neurology 48:1504, 1997.

Firestone S. Challenging the fear industry again. San Diego Tribune, June 11, 1997.

Fisher JC. The silicone controversy—When will science prevail? N Engl J Med 326:1696, 1992.

Fisher JC, Brody GD. Breast implants under siege: An historical commentary. J Long-Term Effects Med Implants 1:243, 1992.

Fisher JC, Potchen EJ, Sergent J. Office communication with breast implant patients: Radiologic and rheumatologic concerns. Perspect Plast Surg 6:(2)79, 1992.

Friis S, Mellemkjaer L, McLaughlin JK, et al. Connective tissue disease and other rheumatic conditions following breast implants in Denmark. Ann Plast Surg 39:1, 1997.

Gabriel SE, O'Fallon WM, Kurland LT, et al. Risk of connective-tissue diseases and other disorders after breast implantation. N Engl J Med 330:1697, 1994.

Gabriel SE, Woods JE, O'Fallon WM, et al. Complications leading to surgery after breast implantation. N Engl J Med 336:677, 1997.

Giltay EJ, Moens HJB, Riley AH, et al. Silicone breast prostheses and rheumatic symptoms: A retrospective follow-up study. Ann Rheum Dis 53:194, 1994.

Goldman JA, Greenblatt J, Joines R, et al. Breast implants, rheumatoid arthritis, and connective tissue diseases in a clinical practice. J Clin Epidemiol 48:571, 1995.

Goldrich SN. Restoration drama: A cautionary tale by a woman who had breast implants after mastectomy. Ms Magazine 16:20, 1988.

Gorczyca DP, Sinha S, Ahn CY, et al. Silicone breast implants in vivo: MR imaging. Radiology 185:407, 1992.

Green S. A woman's right to choose breast implants. The Wall Street Journal, January 20, 1993.

Gumucio CA, Pin P, Young VL, et al. The effect of breast implant on the radiographic detecting of microcalcification and soft-tissue masses. Plast Reconstr Surg 84:772, 1989.

Gutowski KA, Mesna GT, Cunningham BL. Saline-filled breast implants: A plastic surgery educational foundation multicenter outcomes study. Plast Reconstr Surg 100:1019, 1997.

Handel N, Jensen JA, Black Q, et al. The fate of breast implants: A critical analysis of complications and outcomes. Plast Reconstr Surg 96:1521, 1995.

Handel N, Wellisch D, Silverstein MJ, et al. Knowledge, concern, and satisfaction among augmentation mammaplasty patients. Ann Plast Surg 30:1, 1993.

Hart D. The psychological outcome of breast reconstruction. Plast Surg Nurs 16:167, 1996.

Hazelton R. The tort monster that ate Dow Corning. The Wall Street Journal, May 17, 1995.

Hennekens CH, Lee I-M, Cook NR, et al. Self-reported breast implants and connective-tissue diseases in female health professionals. JAMA 275:616, 1996.

Hochberg CH, Perlmutter DL, Medsger TA Jr, et al. Lack of association between augmentation mammoplasty and systemic sclerosis (scleroderma). Arthritis Rheum 39:1125, 1996.

Huber P. Galilio's Revenge: Junk Science in the Courtroom. New York: Basic Books, 1991.

Huber P. A woman's right to choose. Forbes 149:138, 1992.

Implants and the press [editorial]. The Wall Street Journal, January 27, 1992.

Junk science and judges. Review & outlook. The Wall Street Journal, November 8, 1995.

Karns ME, Cullison CA, Romano TJ, et al. Breast implants and connective-tissue disease. JAMA 276:100, 1996.

Kessler DA. The basis of the FDA's decision on breast implants. N Engl J Med 326:1713, 1992.

Kessler DA, Merkatz RB, Schapiro R. A call for higher standards for breast implants. JAMA 270:2607, 1993.

Kolata G. Legal system and science come to differing conclusions on silicone. New York Times, May 16, 1995.

Kolata G. Will the lawyers kill off Norplant? New York Times, May 28, 1995.

Kolata G, Meier B. Implant lawsuits create a medical rush to cash in. New York Times, September 18, 1995.

Laing TJ, Gillespie BW, Lacey JV Jr, et al. The association between silicone exposure and undifferentiated connective tissue disease among women in Michigan and Ohio. Arthritis Rheum 39:S150, 1996.

Macdonald KL, Osteholm MT. A case control study to assess possible triggers and cofactors in chronic fatigue syndrome. Am J Med 100:548, 1996.

McLaughlin JK, Fraumeni JF, Nyren O. Silicone breast implants and risk of cancer? JAMA 273:116, 1995.

McLaughlin JK, Fraumeni JF, Olsen J, et al. Re: Breast implants, cancer, and systemic sclerosis. J Natl Cancer Inst 86:1424, 1994.

McLaughlin JK, Nyrin O, Blot WJ, et al. Cancer risk among women with cosmetic breast implants. A population-based cohort study in Sweden [brief communication]. J Natl Cancer Inst 90:156, 1998.

Noone RB. A review of the possible health implications of silicone breast implants. Cancer 79:1747, 1997.

Park AJ, Black RJ, Sarhadi NS, et al. Silicone gel-filled breast implants and connective tissue diseases. Plast Reconst Surg 101:261, 1998.

Park AJ, Chetty U, Watson ACH. Patient satisfaction following insertion of silicone breast implants. Br J Surg 49:515, 1996.

Park AJ, Walsh J, Reddy PSV, et al. The detection of breast implant rupture using ultrasound. Br J Surg 49:299, 1996.

Peters WJ, Smith DC, Fornasier V, et al. An outcome analysis of 100 women after explantation of silicone gel breast implants. Ann Plast Surg 39:1, 1997.

Petit JY, Le MG, Mouriesse H, et al. Can breast reconstruction with gel-filled silicone implants increase the risk of death and second primary cancer in patients treated by mastectomy for breast cancer? Plast Reconstr Surg 94:115, 1994.

Reed ME. Daubert and the breast implant litigation: How is the judiciary addressing the science? Plast Reconstr Surg 100:1322, 1997.

Risk Assessment of Polyurethane Breast Implants. Rockville, Md.: U.S. Food and Drug Administration, Department of Health & Human Services, July 1, 1991.

Romanelli JN, Solomon G, Silverman S, et al. More on breast implants and connective-tissue diseases. N Engl J Med 332:1306, 1995.

Rose NR. The silicone breast implant controversy: The other courtroom. Arthritis Rheum 39:1615, 1996.

Sanchez-Guerrero J. Autoantibody testing in patients with silicone implants. Clin Lab Med 17:341, 1997.

Sanchez-Guerrero J, Colditz GA, Karlson EW, et al. Silicone breast implants and the risk of connective-tissue diseases and symptoms. N Engl J Med 332:1666, 1995.

Sanchez-Guerrero J, Liang MH. Silicone breast implants and connective tissue diseases: No association has been convincingly established. Br Med J 309:822, 1994.

Schusterman MA, Kroll SS, Reece GP, et al. Incidence of autoimmune disease in patients after breast reconstruction with silicone gel implants versus autogenous tissue: A preliminary report. Ann Plast Surg 31:1, 1993.

Science abdicates [editorial]. The Wall Street Journal, January 9, 1992.

Sergent JS, Fuchs H, Johnson JS. Silicone breast implants and rheumatic diseases. In Kelly WN, et al., eds. Textbook of Rheumatology, 5th ed. Philadelphia: WB Saunders, 1997.

Shiffman MA. Breast implants and cancer. J Natl Cancer Inst 90:248, 1998.

Stossel J. Protect us from legal vultures. The Wall Street Journal, January 2, 1996.

Strom BL, Reidenberg MM, Greundlich B, et al. Breast silicone implants and risk of systemic lupus erythematosus. J Clin Epidemiol 47:1211, 1994.

Taubes G. Silicone in the system. Discover, The World of Science 16:64, 1994.

U.S. Survey clears implants of role in breast cancer. New York Times, November 17, 1997.

Wigley FM, Miller R, Hochberg MC, et al. Augmentation mammoplasty in patients with systemic sclerosis. Data from the Baltimore Scleroderma Research Center and Pittsburgh Scleroderma Data Bank. Arthritis Rheum 35:S46, 1992.

Williams HJ, Wiseman MH. Silicone breast implants in patients with undifferentiated connective tissue disease. Arthritis Rheum 37:S422, 1994.

Wolfe F. Silicone breast implants and the risk of fibromyalgia and rheumatoid arthritis. Arthritis Rheum 38:S265, 1995.

Wong F. A critical assessment of the relationship between silicone breast implants and connective tissue diseases. Regul Toxicol Pharmacol 23:74, 1996.

Woods JE, Arnold PE. Fiction obscures the facts of breast implants. The Wall
Street Journal, April 7, 1992.
What are clinical trials all about? (92-2706). National Cancer Institute, 1992
(800-4-CANCER).

Breast Implant Internet Sites
Frontline
Medical Journal and Study Abstracts on Breast Implants and
Associated Medical Risks

www2.pbs.org/wgbh/pages/frontline/implants/medical/abstracts.html

- Silicone Breast Implants and the Risk of Connective-Tissue Diseases and
  Symptoms (New England Journal of Medicine)
- Breast Implants, Rheumatoid Arthritis, and Connective-Tissue Diseases in a
  Clinical Practice (Journal of Clinical Epidemiology)
- Breast Silicone Implants and the Risk of Systemic Lupus Erythematosus (Jour-
  nal of Clinical Epidemiology)
- Risk of Connective-Tissue Diseases and Other Disorders After Breast Implan-
  tation (New England Journal of Medicine)
- Scleroderma and Augmentation Mammoplasty—A Causal Relationship
  (New Zealand Journal of Medicine)
- Incidence of Autoimmune Disease in Patients After Breast Reconstruction
  With Silicone Gel Implants Versus Autogenous Tissue: A Preliminary Report
  (M.D. Anderson Cancer Center)
- Augmentation Mammoplasty in Patients With Systemic Sclerosis: Data From
  the Baltimore Scleroderma Research Center and Pittsburgh Scleroderma Data
  Bank (Johns Hopkins Medical Institution)
- Silicone Breast Implants and Risk for Rheumatoid Arthritis (University of
  Washington Fred Hutchinson Cancer Research Center)
- Self-reported Breast Implants and Connective-Tissue Diseases in Female
  Health Professionals: A Retrospective Cohort Study (Journal of the American
  Medical Association)

Public Statements Issued by Several Medical Associations After Considering
All the Available Scientific Evidence on the Health Effects

www.pbs.org/wgbh/pages/frontline/implants/medical/positionstate.html

- Statement on Silicone Breast Implants. American College of Rheumatology,
  October 22, 1995
- Laboratory Testing for Monitoring Patients with Silicone Breast Implants.
  College of American Pathologists, Appendix CC
- Silicone Breast Implants and Multiple Sclerosis-like Disorder. National Multi-
  ple Sclerosis Society

Books

www.pbs.org/wgbh/pages/frontline/implants/medical/book.html

- Science on Trial: The Clash of Medical Evidence and the Law in the Breast Implant Case. Marcia Angell, M.D.

Additional Information Links

- Chronology of Silicone Breast Implants
- A Quick Tour
    Address and links to newsletters and breast implants support groups
    Glossary of diseases
    Closing arguments, Gladys Laas case
- Beware: P.R. Implants in News Coverage. Laura Flanders, 1996
- Corporate
    Dow Corning's Disclosure of Breast Implant Complications 1960s-1995
    Silicone: A Brief History
    Products with silicone
- Legal
    Closing arguments
    Readings
    An Epidemiologic View of Causation: How it differs from the Legal. Nancy
        Dreyer, Defense Counsel Journal, January 1994.
    Daubert and Junk Science: Have Admissibility Standards Changed? Nancy
        Miller, Defense Counsel Journal, October 1994.
    Legal System Tries to get a Grip on Upsurge in Mass-Injury Suits. Ben L.
        Kaufman, The Cincinnati Enquirer.
    Taking Daubert's "Focus" Seriously: The Methodology/ Conclusion Dis-
        tinction. Kenneth J. Chesbro.
    Biographies of Lawyers. David Bernick, Stanley Chesley, Richard Lami-
        nack, John O'Qinnn
    Glossary
        Important Legal Terms
- Medical
    FDA Indexing Gateway
    The Federal Judicial Center

Health and Medical Resource Sites

- HealthNews: The Breast Implant Story

    www.healthnet.ivi.com/hnews/9604/htm/implants.htm

- USC Health & Medicine: Reconstructing Lives

    www.usc.edu/hsc/info/pr/hmm/sum97/breast.html

- HealthNews: Follow-Up—Breast Implants Unlikely to Cause Disease

    www.healthnet.ivi.com/hnews/9507/htm/follow2.htm

Australian Sites

- Medical Journal of Australia

    www.mja.com.au/public/issues/sepl6/renwick/renabs.html

- Library
    The British Perspective

    www.mja.com.au/public/issues/sepl6/renwick/renbox2.html

    Silicone Breast Implants: Implications for Society and Surgeons

    www.mja.com.au/public/issues/sepl6/renwick/renwick.html

United Kingdom Sites

- British Medical Journal—Press release and links

    www.bmj.com/bmj/archive/7129/7129p.htm#1a

Abstract
    Risk of connective tissue disease and related disorders among women with
    breast implants: A nation-wide retrospective cohort study in Sweden.
Editorial
    Do silicone breast implants cause connective tissue disease?
Letter
    Media are too eager to link silicone to disease.

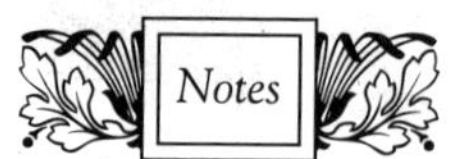

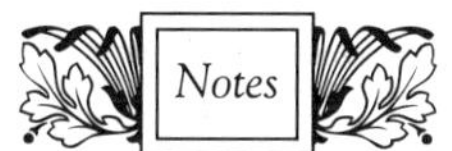

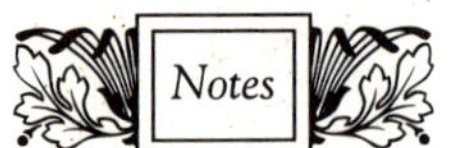

Notes

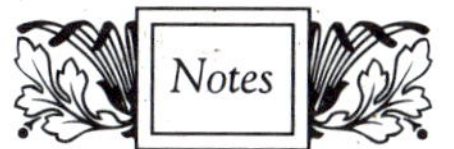

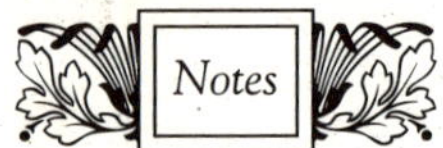

Notes